Curing Our Sick Health Care System

A Solution to America's Health Care Crisis

Robert Gumbiner, M.D.
with Alis Gumbiner

Bloomington, IN 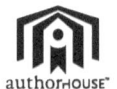 Milton Keynes, UK

authorHOUSE

AuthorHouse™
1663 Liberty Drive, Suite 200
Bloomington, IN 47403
www.authorhouse.com
Phone: 1-800-839-8640

AuthorHouse™ UK Ltd.
500 Avebury Boulevard
Central Milton Keynes, MK9 2BE
www.authorhouse.co.uk
Phone: 08001974150

First published by AuthorHouse 6/29/2006

ISBN: 1-4259-3342-4 (e)
ISBN: 1-4259-3341-6 (sc)
ISBN: 1-4259-3340-8 (dj)

Library of Congress Control Number: 2006904148

Printed in the United States of America
Bloomington, Indiana

This book is printed on acid-free paper.

Contents

ACKNOWLEDGMENTS

A book regarding the cure for our sick and dysfunctional health care system has been on my mind for a long time. For forty years, I have worked my way through solutions to the problem of providing quality, affordable health care on a logical basis. This publication is the product of my experience.

The creation of a book based upon logic, my thoughts, and my experiences was first suggested to me by my daughter, Alis, and culminated in a project based on our discussion, my dictation, and her organization of the first draft of the book. There have been several subsequent edits and rewrites by both of us.

I would like to acknowledge the help extended by my typist, Karen Rasmussen, my research assistant, Danielle Stoumbos, the cover designer, Carmina Padilla and, of course, my daughter, Alis Gumbiner, for her support and effort over the last two years.

Preface

During my career of more than fifty years in health care, first as a practicing physician, then as the creator and manager of a large staff-model HMO, it has been my privilege to witness the change and diversity of the health care system in the United States. This change has been characterized by starts and stops, and blind alleys. There have been some failed attempts to make sense out of what has happened to our health care system and to bring affordable, accessible, quality health care to the long-suffering and long-paying citizens of the United States.

Various well-intentioned efforts have been diverted or sabotaged through the opposition of entrenched enemies of progress and reality. These opposing forces have gained strength through the very mechanism that is being held out as the foundation of the best health care in the world: the fee-for-service, for-profit motive for the provision of health care. Resistance to change was originally spearheaded by doctors in the form of organized medicine through the American Medical Association, who clung tenaciously to the past, imperfect as it was.

The center of the opposition to the improvement of health care delivery has now moved to the more powerful sectors of the health care industry: the prescription drug companies and their allies, for-profit hospitals, and the for-profit health insurance sector of the economy. These forces are much more dangerous to progress, since they are well-financed and are not subject to the ambivalence facing doctors who are trying to make a living while being caregivers. Pharmaceutical and insurance companies are motivated by profit: a motive supported by their investors, shareholders, and management.

Throughout my career, one of my interests has been to travel to various countries, developed, semi-developed, and undeveloped, to investigate their health care delivery systems and their attempts to provide financial support for those systems. These range from the wholly government-sponsored and -controlled systems of the communist (and some socialist) countries, to the semi-socialized systems of Great Britain and Sweden, to systems of partially developed countries.

The observations I include in this book are practical suggestions I have gleaned from more than thirty-five years of health care management and development efforts. My experience includes establishing one of the first group-practice prepayment organizations in the 1960s and guiding its evolution into a combination of a staff-model HMO with independent practice HMOs combined with an innovative health insurance company. As the reader is exposed to my views on the myths and realities of what are generally espoused as "solutions" for our troubled health care delivery system, I anticipate there may be agreement or disagreement. This book is intended to stimulate discussion, provoke thought, present questions, and open a dialogue on realistic health care reform. Be assured that my observations are based on personal attempts to solve many of the problems we face today, making mistakes and false starts, then regrouping and straightening out these problems using logic, not gimmicks.

The precepts of good management, when applied to the delivery of health care, do work. The non-discretionary, non-market-responsive aspects of health care costs have motivated many of the participants in the health care field to focus on wealth accumulation to the detriment of achieving the original goal of managed care: to provide the most care, to the most people, for the least amount of money.

Chapter 1

The Reality of Health Care in the United States

How and Why the Defenders of the Status Quo Are Misleading the Public

Not too long ago, I went to see my doctor for a check-up following a procedure. He took a look at me and said, "Everything looks good, but just to be sure, let's have a scan done." I said, "Wait a minute; we did a scan two weeks ago. Why do I need another scan?" He said, "We'll do it just to be on the safe side. After all, Medicare pays for it."

Sure, Medicare or an insurance company may pay for it today, but I'll be paying for it next year, and the year after, and the year after that. And so will you. Just because a procedure is "paid for" doesn't mean that procedure is free. Someone, somewhere down the road, is paying for it. Yet doctors may order tests, having no idea what those tests cost. Patients submit to the tests and procedures the doctor orders, and all the bills are sent to a third party – Medicare, Medicaid, or an insurance company – that has no control over what is ordered by doctors. And people wonder why health care costs are out

1

of control? Insurance companies operate to avoid risk, not take risk; if their costs go up, so do their premiums.

The basic health care system in the United States is not working and must be fixed. Today, the purchasers of care (physicians) have no motivation to control costs. The users of the service (patients) have little choice in level of service, price, or quality. Those who pay for the service (the government and insurance companies) have minimal control over the utilization and price of services. The only workable political solution to our current health care crisis is universal national health care funded by the federal government. This will give the government the leverage and economy of scale to negotiate successfully with the special interests now exploiting the system.

The United States is the only major developed-industrialized country in the world without a system for the provision of universal national health care for its citizens. Forty-five million people have no health insurance. Millions more are underinsured due to high deductibles and copayments. In addition, millions of people living in rural and low-income inner-city areas, insured or uninsured, lack adequate access to medical practitioners. Providers may not be in the appropriate specialties in the right geographic areas. There is no control over what specialties doctors go into or where they decide to practice, resulting in maldistribution and a misallocation of resources. All of this results in *de facto* underinsurance for many people covered by government programs such as Medicaid and Medicare. It is a myth that this country has the best health care in the world. How can it be the "best" when adequate health care is unavailable to millions of people?

This condition exists despite the fact that health care expenses in the United States represent fifteen percent of the gross domestic product. To make the situation worse, we spend more on health care than any other developed-industrialized nation ($5,267 per capita in 2002).[1]   Yet every time someone broaches the need for national universal health care, politicians and special interest groups put forth myriad objections to why it can't be done.

"We can't afford it," they like to say. Or, "People aren't willing to pay more taxes." This is nonsense. Anything we spend on a national health care program will be *in place of, not in addition to* what is currently being spent by the government, employers, and individuals. Given the amount of waste, minor fraud, and profiteering that occurs throughout our current system, not only can we afford to provide adequate health care to every person in this country, *we can do it for less than what is being spent now.* The secondary costs of people going without basic health care are a decrease in productivity due to an increase in lost sick time plus untreated illnesses that result in expensive hospital care. Then there is the misuse of expensive emergency room treatment because many people have no coverage or care is not readily available. It isn't really an issue of "we can't afford national health care." How can we afford *not* to have universal national health care?

In my opinion, people will pay into a system that guarantees basic health care for everyone. Look at Japan. Look at Sweden. The citizens of these and other developed-industrialized countries are willing to pay for services received, services that provide them with a better quality of life. We have a public highway system, public schools, public utilities, a plethora of public services all paid for with our tax dollars. Should we

---

1 Gerald F.Anderson, Peter S. Hussey, Bianca K. Frogner, and Hugh R. Waters, "Health Spending in the United States and the Rest of the Industrialized World," *Health Affairs,* 24, 4 (July/August 2005).

privatize the police and fire departments, or the military? Why should a basic, non-discretionary service like health care be handled any differently than other essential services?

Opponents of universal health care argue, "If we make health care available to everyone, people will use more services, and it will cost us even more." This is a fallacy. Just because a person has dental coverage doesn't mean she will rush to the dentist. People don't like to go to doctors and dentists, for many reasons. They don't like to be probed and prodded. It takes time away from other activities. Most importantly, the doctor may tell them there is something wrong with them. Availability of care will not lead to over-utilization. On the contrary, the lack of basic care results in increased costs from easily avoided prolonged illnesses, expensive complications, and hospital admissions.

Another myth is, "The American people won't stand for socialized medicine – it will take away their choices and put too much control in the hands of the government." These particular objections are based on two very important misconceptions regarding the role of government and the concept of choice. Government-funded national health care is *not* "socialized medicine." *Socialized medicine* means the government owns and manages all health care facilities – clinics, hospitals, nursing homes, and others – and that all health care personnel are employed on a salary by the government. Government *funded* health care means that the government is the *single payer* of health care. The advantage is that everyone in the country is covered by one large pool of funds, administered by the government. This puts the government in a position to control the costs – not the delivery – of health care by negotiating prices with doctors, hospitals, drug companies, and other suppliers.

Single-payer national health care is not socialized medicine. This is a myth perpetuated by opponents to national health care because they believe "if you can't convince them, confuse them" ("them" being the voters).

These same people like to promote the myth that national health care will mean you can no longer choose your doctor. Remember the television advertisement during the Clinton years with John and Harriet, sitting at the kitchen table, expressing their fear that choice would be taken away? That ad was instrumental in defeating efforts at health care reform under that administration. The reform failed, in part because it offered an overly complicated solution. But it also failed because its opponents knew just which buttons to push. In reality, the idea of choice is illusory. Not everyone chooses his or her doctor today; that choice is limited by recommended insurance company panels, by location, and by the doctor's availability. Even if this weren't true, few people have the knowledge and information they need to find and make an informed choice of physician. When the insurance company gives you a list of participating physicians, what are your options for evaluating the training, judgment, skills, or empathy of a particular doctor?

Another fear the opponents to single-payer health care like to play on is the notion that under a government-funded system, health care will be "rationed." Perhaps it's true that a national health care system will place some limits on what is paid for by the government. But isn't it better for *everyone* to get a basic level of care – medical, dental, pharmaceutical, hospital – than for some people to get a lot of care and millions more to get little or none at all? People today want to pay for Volkswagen coverage and get Cadillac benefits in a health care system. That's simply not realistic.

The opponents to any change in our wasteful, inadequate health-care delivery system can be expected to claim that a national single payer system will "ration" health care and limit freedom of choice. There is, however, an answer to this argument: a two-tier system. The first tier, funded through the federal government, would provide complete health care coverage to every citizen, including doctor care, hospitalization, prescription drugs, mental health treatment, dental, optical, and preventive care. This might entail less "choice" but would involve no out-of-pocket cost. For those individuals who want a greater choice, a second tier system could be offered through government sponsored supplemental coverage (with copayments at the time of service), providing consumers the opportunity to make alternate choices of doctors or venues for care and a wider selection of prescription drug coverage. If you stop paying for the supplemental coverage, you drop back to the no-cost basic plan. National health insurance would thus provide a safety net for all citizens, plus greater choice for those willing to pay more. This is similar to our current options in travel and dining: coach or first class, standard rooms or suites, and counter service or high-end white tablecloth dining.

"We don't need government funded health care – there is plenty of private insurance available." This is another fallacy. This is not only a fallacy; it's a tragic lie. Let's look at the very idea of health "insurance." Insurance is designed as protection against something that *might* happen, like theft, fire, flood, or premature death. Insurance for health care is not really "insurance" – it is prepayment for the inevitable. Everyone will need some kind of health care at some point in his or her life. This is not a "may be"; it is a fact. People are born; they die; and in between, they will experience injury and illness. Yet we're supposed to rely on health care coverage from companies whose very business is based on the notion of "underwriting" – guarding themselves from exposure by underwriting policies with exclusions and limitations of coverage. This means that while most people can buy health insurance, it does not provide true health care coverage. It will include copayments, deductibles, and exclusions that limit access to health care. How do insurance companies deal with increases in health care costs? They simply raise the cost of their insurance premiums or reduce the benefits, putting adequate health care coverage out of reach of millions of Americans.

The only way to provide quality, affordable, health care is to put the responsibility for providing care *and* controlling costs in the hands of the providers, mostly the doctors. Doctors control what patients receive in the way of medical care. Under our current system, doctors are not responsible for the cost of providing care. What I am proposing – in greater detail later in this book – a system paid for by the federal government but run by management-trained doctors and administrators working in groups and paid on salary (as most professionals are). This means reorienting physicians away from their current for-profit motive and educating a segment of the health care profession in management and utilization control. To accomplish this, we need to start early – in medical school – by offering three distinct tracks: clinical (treating patients), research, and management. Changing the incentives for health care providers and reorganizing medical education is the only way to affect the outcome.

"We *have* to charge more because…." The end of this sentence will vary depending on which segment of the health care industry is defending its pricing structure. Doctors cite high malpractice insurance rates. Hospital suppliers fault inflation, and hospitals blame new technology. Drug companies point to research expenditures.

In reality, the rise in health care costs is due to multiple factors, most of which have little or nothing to do with the usual suspects of inflation, market forces, scarce resources, increased demand, or escalating costs such as malpractice insurance rates. Rather, the rapid proliferation of new procedures and new prescription drugs (with ever-increasing advertising spin aimed at the public, and the accompanying pressure on doctors) can be listed as major culprits. No one knows what these new drugs and procedures should really cost, since the true expense of research may be less than the very real cost of competitive marketing and advertising.

In addition, who knows what those doctors in the ever-proliferating list of new subspecialties should earn? Where do we draw the line between personal profit and concern for the common good? The perceived non-discretionary aspect of available health care and the inability to reasonably price the services and products that make up the costs of delivering health care defy the usual process of cost control through "market forces."

There are a lot of fingers being pointed at why health care costs have been increasing by ten to fifteen percent a year and many of the groups facing that pointing finger have ready excuses for why they have to charge high prices. Despite these excuses, the cost of delivering health care simply cannot continue to increase at a twelve percent (plus compounding) annual rate and be paid by U.S. industries, individuals and the government.

The American Medical Association has long supported the notion that because doctors spend many years in medical school, they have a right to expect high incomes. I've been to medical school – it's not that tough. University professors may spend just as many years in school, but they don't generate the same level of income. Physicians have traditionally claimed a right to higher income because they have responsibility for life and death and are on call twenty-four hours a day, seven days a week. This is no longer true. The majority of doctors now work in medical groups or organizations, where they share the responsibility for decisions and on-call duties.

Finally, doctors may protest that malpractice insurance drives up the cost of health care, forcing them to charge more for their services so they can pay their premiums. Yet, is malpractice insurance really the culprit? I'd estimate that eighty percent of malpractice suits are brought against twenty percent of the doctors. We don't need malpractice insurance; we need a system for weeding out bad doctors. Maybe the answer is two strikes (i.e., two malpractice suits), and the doctor is denied the practice of high risk procedures; three strikes, he or she is restricted to working as a medic; four strikes, he or she is out of medical practice altogether.

A favorite argument of the pharmaceutical industry is, "We have to charge more because of all the money we spend on research." They stubbornly point to the cost of research and development (R&D) as a justification for charging high prices for proprietary drugs. But guess what? A large portion of that R&D is paid for through our tax dollars. Much of the research for new drugs is conducted by the National Institute of Health or through government-funded grants to universities or other organizations. What R&D the drugs companies do conduct is treated as a tax-deductible expense, so their real cost is reduced by at least a third through tax advantages. Pharmaceutical companies actually make more in profits each year than they spend on research and development.

The drug companies' spending on advertising is designed to convince consumers that they must have the latest new or improved drug. Many of those drugs are copycats that represent no real improvement over anything already on the market and are only marginally effective or actually harmful.

Advertising and profits: that's what we're paying the large drug companies for as the cost of health care increases each year.

Many people – politicians, lobbyists, and special-interest groups – insist that universal national health care is too complicated, too complex, and too expensive. As a result, we have an ineffectual patchwork of partial solutions – the Medicare Prescription Drug Program, the Patients' Bill of Rights, Health Care Savings Accounts, and catastrophic insurance – that fail to get at the source of the problem. We as a nation have to consider the total scope of both the problem and the solution, keeping the end goal in mind at all times: basic health care for everyone in the U.S. *as a right*, not a privilege. This means utilizing the federal government as a single payer, developing a system to control health care costs, delivery and utilization, and re-educating our health care providers and consumers. Perhaps this sounds impossible. I don't believe it is. As the famous Chicago architect, Lewis Sullivan, once said, "Think no small thoughts."

The goal of bringing the most care to the most people for the least amount of money will never be achieved until the current delivery system changes. Let's stop trying to kill a *few* health care alligators one by one; instead, let's drain the swamp and get rid of *all* the alligators. Redesigning the entire health-care delivery system is the only answer to cost control. Unless we change the way in which we deliver care, we have no chance of controlling the costs resulting from the duplication, waste, and fraud that occur in the fee-for-service structure. As things stand now, the more procedures and tests the doctor orders for a patient, whether or not they are needed, the more money that doctor makes. This arrangement is counterproductive. Our current method of delivering health care must be replaced with a planned system. If we can send a man to the moon, why can't the government plan to provide everyone with adequate health care?

This book addresses not only the need for universal national health care, it also offers my ideas on how we can design an effective, equitable system that provides a basic level of health care to all Americans *for no more than we are paying today.* This would involve a simple but planned system, with one pool of funds offering an economy of scale under the control of a single payer (the federal government). It would reorient health care providers by changing their current objectives and reward system, using the Organized Provider System to motivate health care professionals – existing and future – to work within a new framework for providing quality care to *all* people in the United States.

Chapter 2

A Brief History of Our Dysfunctional System

Sixty years ago, doctors were paid for their services by the consumers of those services, just as you pay your auto mechanic, your barber, or the house painter. I began practicing in 1953, about two years before the federal government introduced the first health "insurance" program for federal employers. During those early years, I had to collect from each patient on his or her way out the door. Half the time, I wasn't able to collect anything. On top of this, I had to market my own practice, as did most doctors. Many evenings, I was volunteering for the Cancer League or the Junior Chamber of Commerce, doing my own public relations. At the same time, my wife was busy with local women's groups or entertaining potential referrals. I was in a solo practice, and that's how it was done. Most doctors worked the same way I did, getting themselves known in the community, attempting to collect their fees for services while recruiting and managing their staff, and struggling to keep afloat financially.

What many people, particularly those who "fear" government involvement in health care delivery, don't realize is that our current health care system grew mostly out of the federal government's decision in the mid-1950s to provide health care for all federal employees. This spurred other employers, as well as unions and state and city governments, to begin offering health "insurance" as a benefit to employees, and the health insurance industry expanded.

The Birth of Managed Care

The federal government also promoted the formation of what were then called Prepaid Group Practice Health Plans, taking the position that any federal employee should be able to access prepaid group practice care if they wanted to. This was because the government bureaucrats knew that a planned, organized system for providing care costs less and is more effective. Kaiser Steel is often credited with establishing one of the first prepaid group practice health plans, during WWII, as a means of providing cost-effective coverage for their employees in Fontana, California. Kaiser essentially created a medical group – with all doctors and other health care providers paid on a salary and working out of a Kaiser clinic – that provided care to Kaiser employees. (Prepaid group practice health care actually started twenty-five or thirty years earlier, with physician programs in the Midwest that provided all the health care for their patients for one set fee per month. The doctors and other health care providers worked for the group, at one facility and on salary, and patients saw only doctors associated with that group.)

The idea behind prepaid group practice health plans was sound: make health care more accessible by charging a set monthly fee per patient, regardless of the amount or kind of treatment received. The fact that health care was prepaid would encourage people to see the doctor before they became seriously ill, which would keep everyone healthier and result in less hospitalization and lower health care costs overall. Because the doctors worked within the group, there was a level of oversight that helped to ensure quality.

The objective behind the system was sometimes referred to as "the three A's" – *affordability, availability, and accessibility*. More importantly, prepaid group health plans provided what was to become a mantra for the managed care industry: the most care for the most people for the least amount of money. The big difference between prepaid health plans and health insurance is that under the former, each individual's health care is paid for on a regular basis, and the assumption is that everyone will use it (including preventive care); the latter gambles on most people never needing to access health care. The group practice prepayment provided complete coverage with a stop loss for the *patient,* while health insurance attempts to avoid risk through exclusions and limitations with a stop loss for the *insurance company.*

The groups that benefited most from prepaid group health plans, initially, were the unions. This was another benefit they could negotiate for their members, a means of providing complete care at a reasonable cost. Then the federal government did the analysis and realized they could save quite a bit of money providing care to *their* employees through these plans. The federal government actively promoted the growth of prepaid plans by offering contracts to medical groups who would provide prepaid, capitated – one payment per month per head – health care to federal employees. They appointed Marie Henderson as a type of czar for the program. She traveled across the country, evaluating individual groups and awarding and monitoring contracts. So the driving force behind prepaid group health plans was the federal government. The state governments and the unions followed along because they had the statistics; they knew what health care cost and how those costs could be controlled.

But there was a downside to the government contract system. Every time Congress pressured the federal government to control health care spending, the feds would cut the rates for the group practice prepayment operations, not the fees paid to doctors in fee-for-service practice. It was the simplest way they could reduce health care expenses. They couldn't control the utilization (volume) or charges by fee-for-service doctors because they had no contracts with individual doctors. But they could reduce payments to prepaid plans, which made it harder for those plans to survive. In the face of our current health care crisis, it is disheartening to realize that sixty years ago we had the beginnings of a full-service, preventative health care system that could have eventually provided care to everyone at a reasonable cost.

During the 1960s and 1970s, health care delivery continued through a mixture of health insurance and some prepayment programs. More and more employers were forced to offer health care coverage to stay competitive in attracting and retaining employees. This coverage was available either through a prepaid program or through traditional indemnity insurance (meaning that the insurer indemnifies you for your health care costs; you go to the doctor or hospital and the insurance company pays the bill based on a claim filed by that doctor or hospital). The problem with the indemnity system was that insurers had no control over the amount and appropriateness of the care and what the doctors or hospitals charged. Insurance companies are not in the business to lose money; they are in the business of avoiding risk. If they incur excessive losses this year, they cover those losses with next year's rate increases, by increasing exclusions, deductions, and co-pays, or by getting rid of the older insured who require more care.

What may have been forgotten by some was the reason Medicare passed in the late 1960s: indemnity health and accident insurance companies were unable to cover people over the age of sixty-five. They could not spread the risk of rising costs, new and expensive tests and procedures, plus the increased liability of older patients, on an individual basis. It was mainly the sick elderly who would buy this expensive elder care coverage, causing what insurers refer to as "adverse selection." Covering only the sick led to insurance company losses and created a financial death spiral.

Although proven more cost effective, the prepaid capitated programs faced attack from several directions. The American Medical Association (AMA) viewed them as a kind of communist plot, the precursors of socialized medicine. American doctors, according to the traditions of the AMA, were not meant to work on salary nor have their fees controlled. The AMA had already fought and lost the battle against fee-for-service group practices, which had undermined organized medicine's view of the "traditional" medical practice, where the physician hangs up a "shingle" and operates as a solo doctor. This doctor might have a partner or two, but a partnership is not an organized medical group. It took the AMA a number of years to accept the Mayo Clinic for membership, because they didn't like medical group practice, even if it was fee-for-service.

Prepaid groups also faced resistance from the community, encouraged by the AMA and organized medicine. Doctors practicing fee-for-service medicine thought their practices were threatened by prepaid groups, and they used their offices as bully pulpits, attempting to influence the views of their patients. Those patients included policymakers such as the mayor and city council members. When I started a prepaid group in 1960, I was considered a maverick or an outlier. One day, my mother went to see her internist, and he confronted her, saying, "How can your son do a thing like this? It's unethical." What *he* was doing – lobbying my mother in the exam room – was unethical. I told her to change doctors! This doctor was exhibiting a common fear that medicine would be "taken over" by prepaid groups, or even the government.

Of course, this doctor was not alone in his fear, which persists today among American physicians. But in reality the fee-for-service physician is fast becoming an anachronism in most developed-industrialized countries. One of my hobbies has always been visiting countries to review their health care delivery and funding systems. By visiting with government officials, doctors, patients, hospital administrators, medical associations, and others, and asking the right questions, I could get a fair idea of how systems were working or not working.

In Finland, the Finnish Medical Association made a deal with the government, requiring all licensed doctors to belong to the Finnish Medical Association. In return, the medical association required that all of its members accept the government-financed patient care and the posted fee schedules. Since all of the Finnish doctors were in the system, there was very little reason for private care to exist. When I asked the president of that medical association if there were any doctors practicing outside the system, he told me that out of several thousand doctors, only six refused to join the system. In answer to my question of how they were able to survive financially, his terse answer was "Wealthy spouses!" The lesson learned was that a national health care system provides tremendous leverage for doctor compliance.

As prepaid group health plans matured, they faced another, internal obstacle: competent management. Doctors simply were not, and are not, trained to manage businesses, particularly in an increasingly competitive atmosphere. Essentially, doctors are trained as advisers. They cannot and do not force anyone to do anything, even if it is in the patient's best interest. The manager's job is to make things happen, give direction, and assure compliance. There is a clear dichotomy between practicing medicine and managing a business. Organized, planned, and capitated prepaid health care appealed to me as a doctor, because I didn't like the problem of being a personal physician while trying to get delinquent patients to pay. Prepayment provided a regular, predictable income for the medical group and allowed us to plan efficiently.

Some doctors in my own medical group didn't like the capitation prepayment program. Out of ten doctors in the original group, maybe one or two understood the concept and embraced the program; the others went along (almost under duress) or quit. One of our physicians, who was a good doctor and understood the concept, eventually left the group because his wife wanted to be prominent in the AMA Auxiliary, and they wouldn't let her in as long as he worked in a prepaid group practice health plan. Ironically, thirty years later, the leadership of the local AMA came to me and asked if I would enroll our doctors in the AMA. (By that time, we had about 400 doctors, and the local AMA membership was down by fifty percent.)

Eventually, the opponents to prepaid plans expanded to include pharmacies and hospitals. In the 1960s, soon after I started a prepaid health plan with our ten-doctor group of half general practitioners and half specialty doctors, we realized that most of our patients didn't have good hospital insurance; they had large copayments, large deductibles, and policy limitations. I believed the doctors held the key to controlling hospital costs, because they were responsible for determining the admission, the length of stay, and the amount and kind of treatment in the hospitals, so I decided that we (the doctors) should pay the patient's hospital bill. It made logical sense. But to do this in a cost-effective way, I had to negotiate rates with local hospitals and, most importantly, deny payment for hospital overcharges and services not received. This was the only way we could assure our patients had access to the hospital care they needed. Attending physicians are in the best position to approve payment, because it is the doctor who orders (or doesn't order) the hospital services.

I can vividly remember a charge for transporting one of our patients within the hospital. We investigated and found that this charge was for moving the patient from his room to the X-ray department on a hospital gurney. That charge was "redlined" (i.e., we refused to pay it). Eventually, our policy became one of adjusting or deleting *all* excessive or inappropriate charges. Since these charges were indefensible, hospitals never challenged us (although they did bad-mouth us throughout the medical community). Monitoring hospital charges resulted in lower costs for our enrollees. As did our use of bulk-purchased, low-cost generic medications – provided to our members at low or no cost – which didn't make us popular with the pharmacies.

Despite all the opposition, prepaid group health plans continued to grow, mainly because the patients accepted and appreciated the concept. They generally liked coming to one place for all their care – medical, dental, pharmaceutical – at a set price. When we first converted to prepaid, our medical group offered the plan, on a voluntary basis, to individual families on our existing patient list, and we enrolled 3,000 people.

From HMO to IPA

By the end of the 1960s, the prepaid industry was trying to find a more appealing, all-encompassing title. "Group Practice Prepayment Organization" is not only a mouthful, it was difficult to sell as a slogan and sometimes difficult to understand, so the name Health Maintenance Organization (HMO) came into being. From its inception, this term was applied to the staff-model prepaid group, in which all doctors and health care providers worked for a salary; they were "on staff" for the prepaid group health program, which collected a monthly fee to provide health care to members.

Meanwhile, the health insurance industry was growing at a rapid rate as more and more employers were encouraged – or mandated by federal legislation – to offer health coverage as a benefit. The problem was, and remains, that insurance companies don't know much about providing health care. Doctors order the care, patients receive the care, and the insurers – as a third party – pay for the care. As "third-party payees," insurers have no real control over the cost or utilization of health care.

As a result, insurance companies were forced to pick and choose, attempting to insure those people who were a lower risk, and avoiding those who were a higher risk, particularly people buying individual policies, but also groups. A good example of this was the elderly. Insurance companies tried, and failed, to insure people over sixty-five years of age. Because of the monthly premium, only the sick elderly enrolled, so the insurers couldn't spread the risk over a large enough group to make it work. Only the government, as the single payer of Medicare, could spread the risk by automatically enrolling everyone, sick and well, over age sixty-five. There was no other way at that time to offer health care coverage to this segment of the population.

The federal government has long had a vested interested in providing the most health care to the most people at the lowest cost. That's why they encouraged the development of group practice prepayment plans in the 1950s. That's why they created Medicare in the 1960s. That's why they supported group practice prepayment plans in the 1970s, through the HMO Act of 1973, and by underwriting the start-up of new group practice prepaid plans. Unfortunately, in this last instance, the federal government underestimated the cost and length of time it took to make these new plans successful, and overestimated the availability of competent management and marketing for those plans. The underfinanced/under-managed syndrome soon caught up with the early federal government-sponsored programs, and most failed.

The Federal HMO Act of 1973 mandated that every employer offering traditional health insurance, and with more than a certain number of employees, had to offer those employees the choice of enrolling in an HMO. At the eleventh hour, just as the act was about to pass, the AMA woke up and recognized the threat this legislation posed to what they saw as the traditional practice of medicine. They managed to insert a clause recognizing the Independent Practice Association (IPA) as a type of HMO. This allowed individual practitioners and medical groups to participate and compete under this new legislation. Otherwise, they risked being displaced by a much more organized and efficient system (e.g., the group practice prepayment organization).

The IPA is exactly what it sounds like: an association of independent physicians. But most independent doctors and doctor groups did not understand the IPA and its pricing mechanism, so they grossly under-priced their overpriced services. Individual doctors and small associations or groups of doctors traditionally, without any management experience or education, ran small, risky businesses and absorbed their losses internally. Without realizing it, they were operating on a type of marginal utility concept. Their fixed costs were in place, and they thought down-time meant excess capacity, so they under-priced the services sold to IPAs as a way of filling unused clinical time. These doctors thought joining the IPA would be a windfall, based on their elastic scheduling, but they didn't know the true costs of their services.

The cost of services provided by individual doctors is actually much higher than the cost of equal-quality services provided by organized medical groups. This is due to the economies of scale when fixed costs such as rent and support staff are shared by several physicians. The organized groups can hire skilled management and share the use of facilities, equipment, and staff. Individual practitioners have to duplicate these fixed costs or do without, which is a wasteful system. What the individual practitioners had going for them was they often were using underpaid employees (family members or partially trained assistants), operating out of substandard facilities, and outsourcing expensive procedures. So they made a living, even though in many instances they were not offering the same quality of care and availability that the staff model HMOs provided.

The result was that the IPA was very lucrative for the IPA promoters and managers who created the associations, recruited the doctors, and signed up the patients. These organizers were getting paid on the basis of providing care equivalent to a quality organized system. But they were buying these services from the independent doctors at discounted rates. The motivating factor for the independent doctors was that they viewed membership in the IPA as added income without the cost of marketing; their fixed costs (staff, facilities, equipment) were already covered, and they had some spare time available. Any money they received from the IPA, even though they undercharged for those services, dropped to the bottom line as added income. Besides, since the independent doctors controlled the utilization and frequency of care, they could take the money without worrying about their availability to patients.

The Death of Managed care

The raw numbers indicated that the IPA-type HMO, on a temporary basis, was more profitable, entailed less risk, and was less management-intensive than the staff model HMO (the prepaid group health plan). It could also be established more quickly, and new markets could be entered at lower cost. As staff model HMOs expanded and moved into new markets, they made use of the IPA model as a way to gain entry into those markets and increase their enrollments. What the HMO operators didn't understand or refused to believe was that the IPA doctors would never support the organization that paid them, and were just using it as a temporary means of marketing their services in a competitive environment. Most of the doctors didn't like the IPA; they didn't want anyone telling them what to do or what to charge. They joined under duress, and they didn't really believe in it. Many of them thought prepayment was a good way to make money without doing much.

Early on, before our medical group was transformed into 100 percent prepaid capitation, we attempted to provide service to capitated payment patients and fee-for-service patients through the same doctors. We found the mixture did not work – and never would – because doctors working on a fee-for-service basis make more money the more frequently they see the patient and the more procedures they order. For the capitated patients, the more the doctors do, the less income per service they receive (remember, these patients or their employers are paying one flat fee per month, no matter how much care they receive). This led to a type of schizophrenia. The doctor was unable to tailor his or her treatment plan to the economic appropriateness of the situation, causing confusion and unhappiness among the doctors. They could never grasp the value of the savings under a capitated plan. If the estimated discount for prepaid was thirty percent less than fee-for-service, this discount for the individual doctor was more than offset by cost savings in marketing, billing, and collecting medical fees, surcharges, and deductibles, and billing the insurance company, plus the adjustment for bad debt. All of these savings could easily exceed that thirty percent difference.

This lack of understanding carried over to the IPA contract doctors, who never really supported the capitated concept and continually attempted to undermine the program by making disparaging remarks in front of the patients while they took the IPA's money. This should be a lesson learned: until fee-for-service is phased out, we will have a misguided guerrilla warfare waged by the very doctors and other health care providers who are being supported by the capitated system. In fact, our original medical group doctors (who had converted by about fifty percent to the capitated health plan) broke up over the idea, championed by a majority of these doctors, that their patients would continue to come to them even if it meant paying for services out of pocket. This idea proved to be untrue; eventually seventy percent of their patients left them to stay with the plan. (See Appendix A.)

As professional managers, trained to look primarily at the bottom line, gradually gained control of the HMOs, they quickly realized the profit difference and tended to de-emphasize the more efficient, better quality staff model in favor of the much more lucrative, albeit disorganized and inefficient, IPA model. Kaiser Permanente, one of the originators of prepaid group health, continued with the staff model concept and gradually took over that part of the market. The dominance of the IPA model was compounded as hospitals and medical associations formed their own IPAs as a means of staying competitive.

Then, the large health insurance companies got into the act. They woke up and realized they were paying doctors on a fee-for-service basis, with no way of controlling costs or utilization. Although they often had a fee schedule, some doctors found ways of getting around that by having patients come back for multiple visits, ordering marginal procedures, or mislabeling procedures to collect a higher fee. The insurers knew that the capitated system – paying doctors on a set fee per patient, per month – was the most cost-effective method of paying for health care. But that meant doctors had to join an HMO or an IPA, which not all practitioners were willing to do. Furthermore, some consumers felt they had the right to see any doctor they wanted, but the insurers couldn't get every doctor organized into a group. So the insurance companies invented the Preferred Provider Organization (PPO).

Under the PPO, doctors agree to take a discount off their regular fee schedule for the insurance company enrollees in the PPO. The problem with that is the fee schedule is usually inflated to begin with, so a twenty percent discount off a fee that is fifty percent higher than it should be does not really mean much. Also, the PPO's management (the insurance company) still has no way of controlling utilization, multiple referrals, repeat visits, or duplicated tests and procedures. What the PPO does do is make some people happy because they think they're getting a wider "choice" of doctors.

Many of the people who founded, managed, and controlled the IPAs eventually sold them to established insurance companies, usually at a significant profit. Most of these insurers have moved back to the fee-for-service claims-made method of payment with which they are familiar, and have largely discontinued the capitation rate system that had served to control costs under the HMO model. Instead, these insurance companies attempt to control costs through a system that makes the patient's primary physician a kind of gatekeeper, responsible for referrals to specialists and other physicians. This becomes a type of prior authorization, but not a very good one. It is a bad system. Primary care physicians (mostly internists and/or family practitioners) are not equipped to act as gatekeepers; they are not trained for it. They are not managers; they do not like confrontation, and they do not like the system. Doctors are advisors, not managers. They do not want to be responsible for saying to a patient: "You don't need to see a specialist; I can take care of this." Most importantly, the prior authorization system is inconvenient for the patient, causes delays and extra visits, and gives managed care a negative image.

The core idea behind managed care – that the HMO, rather than the individual physician, would be responsible for the quality, accessibility and availability of health care – virtually disappeared. Larger insurance companies bought up smaller HMOs, buying the membership (but not the concept) and turning HMO members back into insurance company clients, with their health care managed by the limited insurance company mentality.

The final deathblow to the HMO was dealt by the vilification of the very term "Health Maintenance Organization" which, largely through the efforts of the medical establishment's spin artists, came to represent poor quality, rationing, and a lack of concern for the patient. The irony is that this negative spin, fueled by prejudicial advertising and publicity supported by the AMA, insurance companies, and hospitals, were not really justified until after the true HMO was replaced by the insurance company IPA and eventually by managed care. Insurance companies now apply the term "managed care" to something that is anything but.

All of this has led to a poorly organized system of health care, funded through multiple sources and managed primarily by companies that know little about health care, less about health care delivery, and have only minimal control over costs. Most care is provided by fee-for-service doctors, contracting with insurance companies while working independently or in groups with little or no oversight. The concept of "the most care for the greatest number of people at the lowest cost" has been set aside by a large portion of the health care industry. Instead, citizens of the United States – one of the largest, wealthiest, most technologically advanced countries in the world – receive their health care through a bizarre patchwork of delivery systems, funded through a complex mix of government, employer, and individual payments.

A large number of these citizens have no health care coverage at all; they are uninsured, or health care is not available where they live and work. Or, what insurance is available and affordable is relatively useless due to large copayments and deductibles. But people *must* get care. When the cost of this care is not covered by health insurance or other privately funded programs, there's only one source left: the federal government or government subdivisions.

The Government's Role in Health Care

I find it somewhat ironic that opponents to universal single-payer health care use the specters of "big government" and "higher taxes" as a rallying cry to drum up support. The federal government has a long history of financing health care: for its employees, for the military, for citizens eligible for certain entitlement programs, through tax cuts to employers, and through subsidies for hospitals and emergency rooms. I estimate that close to one half of all health care dollars come from the government at some level.

Government employees at the federal, state, county, and municipal levels, including the employees of school districts and public colleges and universities, receive health care as part of their employment benefits, funded by tax dollars. Also funded by tax dollars is health care for military dependents, the Veteran's Administration (VA), and the prison systems. The VA alone treats 5.2 million patients annually, with seventy million people (veterans and their families) eligible for VA benefits.[2] All told, this tax-supported health care may serve sixty million people or more, a number roughly equivalent to the population of France.

It is also ironic that many government employees – including those of the Veterans Administration (VA) and the Congress –

---

[2] "Back in the Pink: The VA health care system outperforms Medicare and most private plans," *The Washington Post National Weekly Edition*, August 29-September 4, 2005, 29. Also, data from the Veteran's Administration at *www.va.gov*.

are served by what are essentially staff model health maintenance organizations. Most members of Congress get treatment for serious illness at the clinics and hospitals of Walter Reed and Bethesda, from military medical group doctors working on salary. The VA has more than 300 government-owned hospitals and nursing homes, separate from the government-owned military clinics and hospitals available to active military personnel and their dependents. Prisons have doctors and dentists on site and on staff to care for inmates. Tellingly, many fee-for-service doctors send their own family members with serious or complicated illnesses to medical school centers, another type of staff model HMO.

Then there are the people covered by government-funded health care programs – Medicare, Medicaid, and SCHIP (State Children's Health Insurance Program). There are roughly forty-one million people in the United States covered by Medicare. Medicaid is available to more than fifty million people. SCHIP offers health care coverage to about four million children from low-income families.[3] Allowing for seven million people with dual coverage (low-income seniors covered by Medicaid in addition to Medicare, and the totally disabled who have access to both), there are approximately eighty-eight million individuals receiving some form of health care through these government programs.

Medicare, which is essentially universal single payer health care for all citizens over sixty-five years of age, was enacted in the late 1960s under President Lyndon Johnson's Great Society Program. This is comprehensive health care with the exception of outpatient prescription drugs and

---

[3] Kaiser Family Foundation, "Medicare at a Glance, March 2004; "The Medicaid Program at a Glance," January 2004; "SCHIP Program Enrollment: June 2003 Update," December 2003. Available at www.kff.org.

other essential services. Most estimates indicate that more than fifty percent of the costs for health care services in the United States are for people over age sixty-five. (As an aside, it has always seemed to me discriminatory that we provide health care coverage to citizens over sixty-five and deny the same coverage for the tax-paying citizens under sixty-five.)

The Medicare population will grow significantly as life expectancies increase and the seventy-five million members of the baby boom generation eventually join Medicare. In another twenty years, we may have 100 million people covered by Medicare alone. That will be 100 million voters over the age of sixty-five. Each one of these voters will be represented by at least one other voter – probably an adult child – who would be forced to contribute directly to the health care costs of these seniors with a decrease in Medicare. We end up with roughly 200 million voters out of a U.S. population of about 300 million who will be financially affected by federal health care programs. And they will vote. No wonder politicians regard Medicare legislative change as the "third rail," not to be touched.

Medicare is funded through the Social Security Administration, which in turn is funded through a payroll deduction from working people. Medicare Part A is a hospital insurance program with a deductible; Medicare Part B covers physician and outpatient hospital care with a twenty percent copayment. Medicare does not cover non-hospital prescription drugs, even with the so-called new Medicare Prescription Drug Program. (This is essentially a drug discount program, which raises the question: a discount off of what – unconscionably high prices? the highest retail rate?) Nor does Medicare cover dental and optometry, nor provide much in the way of preventative medicine such as immunizations and routine examinations. Psychiatric care is not included, and home care is extremely limited. Long-term nursing home coverage is excluded. Seniors end up having to buy some form of supplemental insurance (if they can afford or find it) or turn to Medicaid if they are indigent.

Medicaid (Medi-Cal in California), government-funded health insurance for the poor, was enacted as an afterthought at the same time as Medicare. It is funded by the federal and the individual state governments, through a fifty-fifty matching program. The level of services offered through Medicaid is determined by each state, provided the state covers basic doctor and hospital services, resulting in more coverage in some states and less in others. For example, in a large, relatively wealthy state like California, Medicaid covers doctor care, hospitalization, dental, pharmaceutical, and psychiatric care. In smaller, poorer states, less care is covered.

The result of this state-by-state program was and is a disaster. Eligible people seeking care moved from low-coverage states to high-coverage states. The elderly in need of long-term nursing care (which is very expensive) gave away or spent down all their assets to qualify for Medi/Medi, a combination of Medicaid and Medicare for the elderly poor. The cost of Medicaid and the number of people covered are now larger than those figures for the Medicare population. The Medicaid cost for some states has threatened to bankrupt them. Mississippi's Medicaid costs exceeded the whole state budget. New York, with one of the most generous Medicaid programs in the country, spends $44.5 billion annually, or $10,600 for each of the 4.2 million people enrolled in the program.[4]

---

[4] Clifford J. Levy and Michael Luo, "New York Medicaid Fraud May Reach Into Billions," *New York Times,* July 18, 2005. Available at www.nytimes.com.

Strangely, while the AMA (aided by their friends in the Health Insurance Association of America) vigorously and desperately fought to prevent the enactment of Medicare, having lost that battle, then made a switch. The AMA and the HIAA supported Medicaid, mainly because the doctors didn't expect to take care of poor people anyway, and the health insurance companies saw no monetary value in trying to sell insurance to the poor. Neither group viewed this segment of the market as profitable. In fact, eligible Medicaid individuals living in the inner city and rural areas today lack access to medical providers because the majority of doctors choose to practice in higher-income urban areas. This results in a lack of sufficient health care services in the low-income inner city, as well as the poor rural areas. So, although some individuals are eligible for Medicaid, they may be *de facto* not covered because of the lack of available services.

There is no way out of this rapidly increasing problem – an expensive entitlement program that fails to serve the people who need it most – other than to merge Medicare and Medicaid into one federal program. The current problems facing Medicaid highlight the mistake of a using a patchwork of state-supported programs. The catastrophic cost of having one unevenly funded program (Medicaid), as the insurer of last resort for long-term nursing care, may ultimately bankrupt the program. A Medicare/Medicaid merger would at least spread the risk and expense of providing long-term care to over eighty million people. (Universal health insurance would spread it over nearly 300 million people in the United States by including even more non-users.) Another part of the solution to the problem of access to care – the Organized Provider System and the reorganization of the educational system for doctors, nurses and other health care providers – will be dealt with later in this book.

Chapter 3

Why Small Reforms Won't Help Big Problems

It's hard to open a newspaper these days without seeing another story about escalating health care costs. A lot of fingers have been pointed at the pharmaceutical industry, malpractice insurance costs, hospital fees, and fraudulent billing practices. All of these may contribute to rising costs, but the basic problem is in the system itself.

The True Cost of Health "Insurance"

Regardless of the billions of dollars spent by the government, the basis of our health care system is private insurance. The cost of this insurance may be paid by a government entity or private employer (as a job benefit), through a union (partially funded by union dues), or directly out of the individual's pocket. Approximately 163 million people in the U.S. have some form of what is considered privately funded health insurance, which may be through traditional health and accident insurance companies (as indemnity coverage or through a PPO), an IPA, or an HMO.[5]

---

[5] Kaiser Family Foundation and eHealthInsurance, "Update on Individual Health Insurance," August 2004. Available at *www.kff.org*.

This private health insurance system is bloated with waste and duplicate expenses. About five percent of the insurance premium goes to processing claims, and approximately twenty-five percent goes to administration and competitive marketing. The private insurers spend billions of dollars each year advertising and marketing their programs. Plus, since these insurers are in the business to make money, there's another six to ten percent of the premium that represents profit to the insurer. What we have is a health care system that has inserted a third party, the insurance company, between the provider of the service (the doctor and hospital) and the consumer of that service (the patient) at a cost increase of at least forty percent. How do I know this? Because, in addition to running a staff-model HMO and an IPA, I founded and operated a health and accident insurance company, a life insurance company, and a worker's compensation company.

Here's how this system works (or doesn't, depending on your point of view). Health care insurance companies offer a variety of plans with different levels of coverage. They employ a marketing department to advertise those plans, a sales force selling directly to the group and individual purchasers, and a large back-office staff to review claims and make payments. Large, established insurance companies may spend as much as thirty percent of gross revenue on these functions. A smaller insurer or someone new to the market may be spending fifty percent or more on marketing and administration alone. In addition, a new insurance company may be required to hold up to eighty percent of gross revenue in reserve against future claims. This is at the front end.

The cost of actually paying out on claims is something the insurer has little real control over. The patient goes to a doctor; the doctor examines the patient, prescribes a treatment or performs a procedure, and submits a claim for payment. The patient may go to multiple doctors for the same complaint and/or diagnostic tests. Each doctor may order additional tests, procedures, and prescription drugs. The insurer has no control over these actions. Private insurance is simply fee-for-service medicine with a monolithic (and expensive) middleman. As the cost of treatment claims increases, the insurance company simply passes that cost along to the consumer in the form of increased premiums or higher deductibles, larger copayments, and more limitations.

Each year, the cost and parameters of any given program change. The employer, employee, or independent purchaser must spend a considerable amount of time reviewing and comparing various plans to select one offering the best mix of price and coverage. So, there is an additional cost of time spent reviewing the options, plus the cost of forgoing certain kinds of coverage (dental, pharmaceutical, preventative) in an effort to keep premiums affordable. In some cases, the presentation of coverage is so confusing and convoluted that even an insurance actuary would have a hard time understanding the policy.

Employers have to make a profit to stay in business, so they typically deal with increases in health insurance premiums by: a) buying policies that provide less coverage overall; b) passing the cost along to employees in the form of higher deductibles and copayments; or c) laying off employees with chronic conditions or those in older age groups to keep the total health insurance bill at a reasonable level. The number of people under the age of sixty-five covered by employer-sponsored plans dropped from sixty-seven percent in 2001 to sixty-three percent in 2003, and to sixty percent in 2005.

In 2005, the average cost of an employer-sponsored premium for a family of four was $10,088 per year (up from $7,954 in 2002). The employee's share of that $10,088 per year premium was $2,713, with annual deductibles averaging $561 per year.[6] The average employee, with a spouse and a couple of kids, is paying more than $3,000 a year toward health care, even with employer-sponsored health insurance.

Most people with health care coverage are paying far more than they realize in deductibles and out-of-pocket expenses. When they don't have coverage, or that coverage is reduced by exclusions and limitations, they may be paying medical fees for doctor and hospital care at a rate far higher than that negotiated by insurance companies for the same service.

As of 2004, employment benefits represented twenty-nine percent of worker compensation; between 2000 and 2004, the cost of benefits rose to twenty-four percent of workers' income, while wages increased by only fifteen percent.[7] The major reason for the increase in the cost of total benefits, which indirectly decreased worker pay, was the increase in health care costs. The cost of insurance premiums is increasing every year: eleven percent in 2001, thirteen percent in 2002, fourteen percent in 2003, eleven percent in 2004, and nine percent in 2005.[8] When one considers the effect of compounding (i.e., thirteen percent on eleven percent, fourteen percent on thirteen percent), it is even more expensive.

---

[6] Kaiser Family Foundation, "2005 Employer Health Benefits," September 15, 2005. Available at *www.kff.org*; Milt Freudenheim, "Increases in Health Care Premiums Are Slowing," *The New York Times*, May 27, 2004. Available at *www.nytimes.com*.

[7] Kaiser Family Foundation, "Health Care as an Employee Benefit," June 25, 2004. Available at *www.kff.org*.

[8] Jonathan Weisman, "Sick About Health Care Costs," *Washington Post Weekly*, June 7-13, 2004, 29; Kaiser Family Foundation, "2005 Employer Health Benefits." Available at *www.kff.org*.

Barriers to Access

Rising premiums, reduced benefits, and cost-shifting to the individual have created a critical barrier to accessing health care. People are discouraged from seeking health care when they need it, which is before illness becomes severe. People might resist going to the doctor, even though they have health insurance, because there is a $50 copayment for the doctor visit. The unspoken reason is "I want to make sure I am $50 sick before I go see the doctor and pay $50." By the time a patient figures out that he is "$50 sick," he may require hospitalization; now the cost is no longer $50, but $1,600 a day or more. Perhaps the doctor orders a prescription medicine that is not covered or requires a $35 copayment, but the patient waits until payday to fill this prescription. Or the patient fills only half of the ordered prescription, to save money, resulting in a sicker patient who later requires more expensive treatment.

Copayments and deductibles create a barrier to early treatment and limit affordability, preventing people from accessing the care they need, when they need it. They dissuade people from seeking early or preventive care, which could keep them from getting seriously ill in the first place. Think about it: pushing more cost onto the consumer at the time of service may reduce costs to the insurance company in the short term but, in my view, this practice may cost much more in the long term.

Preventive care can greatly reduce overall health care costs. Regular check-ups and immunizations, seeking treatment before an illness becomes acute, and taking the drugs prescribed to treat illness at its beginning stages are all necessary in keeping health care costs down. Large deductibles, copayments, expensive pharmaceuticals, lack of appropriate insurance coverage, and lack of availability of services all create roadblocks to effective health care in the United States.

The Cost of the Uninsured and the Underinsured

More people than we realize fall into a large and largely under-measured group that I call the "under-insured." According to statistics, these people do have health insurance, but the deductibles and copayments may be so large ($2,000 or more each year) that this "insurance" is virtually useless except in catastrophic circumstances where the costs may be considerable. This is the wrong way to go. Besides, these unfortunates – lacking the discount leverage of Medicare or group insurance – may be paying "full" rates; as much as forty percent more than the rates negotiated by insurers.

Many people are further underinsured because they are only *partially* insured; they lack coverage for certain essential services such as dental, optometry, and prescription drugs. In short, the "bicuspid (dental), bifocal (eye care), and bicarbonate (prescription drugs)" are excluded. These services, when combined with doctor care, constitute traditional, ambulatory health care. Without them, a person lacks full health care coverage. What is the purpose of health insurance if the contract with the provider does not result in care? How can you get well without drug coverage, and how healthy are you if you cannot chew? If you cannot see or you have no teeth, you may not be able to work.

This is one of the main reasons health care costs are increasing: people are underinsured, so they wait until they are seriously ill to access health care through their health insurance. The size of this group – the underinsured – has not, to my knowledge, been measured. It includes people with high deductibles and multiple insurance exclusions; it also includes those on Medicare and Medicaid. Medicare provides health care coverage – doctors and hospitalization – to forty-one million Americans, thirty-five million of whom are over the age of sixty-five. Many of these people, particularly the elderly, require some form of long-term care. Because long-term, non-critical care is not covered by Medicare (or most insurance programs), we often end up warehousing seniors and the chronically ill in expensive hospitals and substandard nursing homes.

Medicare recipients are also underinsured due to the lack of prescription drug coverage. Recent programs have done little to alleviate this problem. The so-called Medicare Reform approved in 2003 created a complex system that will do little to lower the cost of prescription drugs. Most seniors take anywhere from six to ten drugs at any given time, costing as much as $600 per month or more. How does somebody choose between a needed prescription and paying the rent? Considering that thirty-seven percent of Medicare recipients have an income below 150 percent of the federal poverty level, this is a very real problem.[9] If these people don't take the drugs they need to prevent illness, they may end up in an expensive hospital or, worse, in intensive care at $3,000 a day or more.

Even if we can't quantify the extent of underinsurance in this country, we do know how many people are without any form of health care insurance: forty-five million at last count (sixty-one million including children). Contrary to popular belief, these are not unemployed layabouts. Eighty percent of people without health insurance are employed; they are the "working poor."[10] A large portion of the remaining twenty percent may have had health insurance at some point in the last two years, but lost it when they changed jobs or were laid off.

---

[9] Kaiser Family Foundation, "Medicare Fact Sheet: Medicare at a Glance," March 2004 Available at www.kff.org

[10] Institute of Medicine Task Force, "Uninsured in America," The Toledo Blade, July 4, 2004. Available at www.toledoblade.com

(This highlights another big problem with our current form of health care: coverage tied to employment.)

The uninsured paid about 32.6 billion dollars out of their own pockets for health care in 2004. What they are unable to pay represents "uncompensated care" on the part of hospitals and emergency rooms, an amount estimated at 40.7 billion dollars in the U.S.A. in 2004. Most of this cost is paid by our government.[11] Unfortunately, what the uninsured do pay out of pocket constitutes an overcharge compared to what is paid by insurance companies for the same services.

With or without insurance, an estimated one in seven families in the United States reported having problems paying medical expenses in 2003. Two-thirds of these people actually had health insurance. Thirty percent did not fill a prescription due to cost; about twenty-five percent delayed treatment for financial reasons.[12] Whenever health care becomes inaccessible due to out-of-pocket expense, the result is more severe sickness at an even higher cost of treatment. Or people get no treatment at all. An estimated 18,000 people die each year because they lack health insurance and cannot get the necessary medical treatment.[13]

The lack of the three critical components in providing health care – affordability, accessibility, and availability – is what leads to increased health care costs. Availability is particularly critical for those fifty million poor people eligible for Medicaid. What the government often ignores in funding health care programs is physical accessibility. Residents of

---

[11] Kaiser Family Foundation, "The Cost of the Uninsured," May 10, 2004. Available at www.kff.org.

[12] Reuters AlertNet, "U.S. Families struggle with Medical Debt," July 1, 2004. Available at www.kff.org.

[13] Institute of Medicine Task Force, "Uninsured in America." Available at www.kff.org.

the inner cities and sparsely populated rural areas lack access to health care services. Not enough doctors practice in these areas, and medical services aren't available at times when Medicaid recipients, the working poor, can get to them (such as evenings and weekends). An hourly worker can't afford to take time off work to go to the doctor, and may lack transportation. Try taking two sick kids to the doctor on public transportation! Medicaid recipients represent another large group of people who are underinsured due to lack of coverage and lack of access to timely medical care. Like others who are underinsured, they wait to seek treatment in hospital emergency rooms.

Health care is often "unavailable" in other ways. Some doctors don't want to see Medicaid or Medicare patients because the government sets limits on how much will be paid for specific services, or because the patients are difficult to work with, due to cultural differences. Many doctors don't want to work in the low-income inner-city or rural areas because it limits their own income, and they don't live there. Other doctors choose to go into high-priced specialties, resulting in overspecialization in areas such as surgical subspecialties and an undersupply of internists and general practitioners (in 2000, only thirty percent of physicians in this country were practicing as generalists or internists).[14] Approximately thirty-six million Americans report that they can't obtain health care – even with insurance – because doctors don't accept their insurance or facilities aren't available in their area.[15]

---

[14] American Medical Association, Physician Characteristic and Distribution (Chicago: AMA, 2001)

[15] Kaisernetwork, "Access to Care Problems Affect 36M U.S. Residents, NACHC Report Finds," March 30, 2004. Posted at www.kff.org.

The Role of the Doctor

For some reason, the debate over how to "fix" our ailing health care system rarely touches on the role of the doctor. This is despite the fact that doctors are the only people with control over the cost of delivering health care; doctors order the tests, the drugs, and the treatments, and control the volume or utilization of services. The insurance companies simply pay for the services ordered by doctors (provided those services are covered by the patient's policy).

Unfortunately, some doctors actively contribute to rising health care costs through various forms of major and minor fraud. They might input the wrong code when filing a claim for a procedure (intentionally or unintentionally) and collect more than the insurer would have paid for the procedure that is actually performed. For example, a "consultation" pays more than a regular office visit. The doctor may re-order procedures, order extra procedures, put the patient in the hospital when it's not necessary, and order tests that aren't really needed. All of these actions represent claims filed with the insurance company, Medicare, or Medicaid, and serve to drive up the cost of health care. After all, doctors are only human; under our fee-for-service system, the more they do, the more money they make.

The fault is in the fee-for-service system, a throwback to the 19th century. The Department of Health and Human Services estimated fraud and abuse in Medicare and Medicaid billing alone at close to one billion dollars in 2003.[16] BlueCross/BlueShield has announced plans to launch

---

[16] Kaisernetwork, "Fraud, Abuse in Medicare and Medicaid Could Exceed Government Tracking Figures," April 20, 2004. Posted at www.kff.org.

a national task force investigating an estimated fifty billion dollars in fraudulent claims on the part of doctors.[17] The federal government's General Accountability Office estimates payment of fraudulent claims at ten percent of annual national Medicare spending.[18]

Many doctors allege that they have to run multiple tests to prevent getting sued by the patient. To my mind, this is simply an excuse, stemming from a lack of diagnostic competence or the inability to make a decision. You don't run test panels on everything; that is a waste of time and resources. Granted, things are more complicated today. The doctor has more tests to think about and a plethora of diagnoses and treatments to consider, but experience and confidence should lead a doctor to proceed in a logical manner. The approved protocol is to select one or two presumptive diagnoses based upon a careful history and physical, and then order only those lab and diagnostic procedures that will confirm or eliminate those diagnoses. This is why most sophisticated medical centers have developed a protocol for diagnosis and treatment. This helps get at the root of the problem of waste and duplication.

The Malpractice Myth

I'm not pointing a finger at doctors in general. The majority of doctors are caring, competent professionals who sincerely want to do what is best for the patient. But as with other professionals, such as lawyers, accountants, and architects, there are some who have poor judgment, are insensitive, may have poor patient rapport, or

---

[17] Kaisernetwork, "BlueCross BlueShield Assocation to Launch National Task Force to Address Health Care Fraud," April 20, 2004. Posted at www.kff.org.

[18] Clifford J. Levy and Michael Luo, "New York Medicaid Fraud May Reach Into Billions," New York Times, July 18, 2005. Available at www.newyorktimes.com.

are careless and do not keep up with the latest developments in the field. Malpractice insurance is used as an excuse for raising fees. This is a fallacy. Malpractice really isn't a widespread problem. A recent study showed that fifty-three percent of all malpractice settlement payments are made by five percent of doctors.[19]

In my experience (over forty-five years of hiring and managing physicians), I would say that eighty percent of malpractice claims are filed against twenty percent of doctors. We don't need malpractice insurance; we need to get rid of the problem doctors. Not all people who graduate from medical school should become practicing physicians or remain in clinical medicine, treating patients. I can remember vividly errors by board certified specialists that led to liability. There was a qualified OB specialist who was so busy watching a televised football game that he didn't check the fetal monitor during labor and, when the baby got into trouble, blamed it on the nurse. Then there was the doctor who said he told the patient to return to see a cardiologist because of an abnormal EKG, but he did not put a note in the patient's chart. Guess what? The patient did not return and died at an elevation of 8,000 feet (on a ski slope) one year later. Would that patient have been more or less likely to go skiing, knowing that he had an abnormal EKG? With a blank chart, our company lost that malpractice case.

Although difficult to achieve with the medical profession locking their horns around their wounded colleagues, the following system might even be welcomed by some doctors seeking a way out of the malpractice morass; it certainly would save a lot of money, pain, and suffering. This is my suggestion: those doctors who have a malpractice claim lodged

---

[19] Public Citizen, "Fifth Vote on Malpractice Bill Follows Poor Health Care Quality Findings," May 12, 2004. Available at www.citizen.org.

against them (many of which are valid) should first be given a warning. The second malpractice claim should prohibit them from performing high-risk procedures such as obstetrics and surgery. After a third claim, that provider should be assigned to a mid-level status such as medic. If there are problems at that level – after retraining and reorientation – that doctor should be denied medical licensing in any sector of the health care field. Like it or not, there are doctors who are just not very good, or whose skill level has deteriorated since they graduated medical school thirty years ago.

Another major cause of malpractice litigation is the general public's dislike of the medical profession as a whole. In the fifteen years that I actively practiced, I was never sued, because I always talked to the patients. I worked hard, and my patients and their families saw me coming and going, all night long. I would tell them: "I tried as hard as I could, we did everything, but we just couldn't save your father." I called in consultants; I kept the patient's family informed of what was being done. And they saw that. But if a doctor is negligent, doesn't show up, is arrogant, has little empathy toward the patient and the family, then the patient or the family is going to sue because they're angry and want to punish that doctor. From their point of view, the doctor treated them badly and, to make matters worse, overcharged them in the process.

Believe me, the problems of the doctor who told the patient to return and forgot to note it in the chart (and the patient died), and the OB doctor who was watching television in the hospital while the monitor indicated that the fetus was in trouble, were real cases. Both of these physicians were board certified in their specialty and may still be practicing today in the fee-for-service sector.

Physician oversight is critical in reducing the incidence of malpractice. Doctors working in a team are less likely to make mistakes. Here is another argument for a single-payer health care system run through organized provider groups: there is a significant economy of scale achieved through the purchase of malpractice insurance for a large group of physicians. In the staff model HMO I managed for more than thirty years, we maintained malpractice coverage for 700 professionals (doctors, dentists, and pharmacists) with a three million-dollar deductible, overall. In addition, we had our own claims prevention and adjustment system, employing an attorney and claims advisors. These people followed up on any complaint or alleged problem and corrected or settled it before it got into litigation. We terminated professionals who were suit-prone. We spent about one million dollars a year on this claims prevention program, resulting in an annual overall cost of less than $5,000 per professional. Taking into account a relatively low premium per doctor, plus a small piece of the three million-dollar deductible, this equals a fraction of what independent physicians pay. The ability to partially self-insure, eliminate problem health care providers, and negotiate insurance premiums resulted in huge savings in the cost of malpractice insurance, a cost that is all too often passed along to the consumer under our current, disorganized system.

Drugs and Technology: How much do we really need?

Every day, pharmaceutical representatives visit doctors' offices to make their pitch on the latest wonder drug and hand out free samples. Then the drug companies spend millions of dollars advertising the latest drug, regardless of whether it is more effective than something already on the market. Through direct consumer advertising, the public is led to believe that drugs will cure anything, and doctors do not necessarily argue with that perception.

Unfortunately, many doctors conclude a visit by giving the patient a prescription: "Take this, see how you get along, call me, or come back for a check-up." While this may provide a solution for the doctor, it may not be in the best interest of the patient. Maybe the patient needs a different diet, an exercise program, a reduction in stress, or a change in lifestyle. In addition, patients are convinced by pharmaceutical advertising to put pressure put on their physicians. What can a doctor do for the person with incurable, degenerative arthritis, who demands that new, widely advertised cure? Prescribe it. It doesn't cost the doctor anything.

Unfortunately, many doctors have no idea what the prescription is going to cost the patient; it may not be covered by insurance, or it may require a $50 deductible. Individual expenditures on prescription drugs increased about fifty percent between 1998 and 2002. Drug expenditures represented almost two percent of individual income in 2002.[20] Regardless of whether the drug is paid for by the patient or the insurer, the overuse of expensive brand-name prescription medicines contributes to the rising cost of health care. New drugs and procedures, particularly those marketed directly to the consumer, are two reasons health care costs are not market responsive.

The high price of pharmaceuticals, according to the drug companies, is justified by the cost of research and development (R&D). This is nonsense. Most of the research into new drugs is underwritten by the government, through the National Institute of Health (NIH) or by various grants to academic centers or other private and public sources. Yet we pay several times more for drugs developed in this country with our tax

---

[20] Boston University School of Public Health, "Study on Prescription Drug Costs," The Boston Herald, July 15, 2004. Available at www.bostonherald.com.

dollars than consumers pay in other countries. Whatever R&D the drug companies do pay for (directly) in the U.S. may be reduced by tax credits from the federal government. The high price we pay for pharmaceuticals cannot be due solely to the cost of manufacturing the drugs, because most of the same prescription drugs are available for much less in Canada, Europe, India, and Mexico.

A good portion of what we pay for drugs is due to the millions of dollars the pharmaceutical industry spends each year to convince us, through mass-media advertising and pressure on doctors, that we need those drugs. In 2000, drug company spending on R&D increased by thirteen percent; advertising expenses increased by thirty-two percent.[21] Drug company profits represent a big chunk of the cost of prescription medicines. Pharmaceutical companies make more in profits than they spend on R&D.[22] Without the advertising, marketing, and administrative costs, plus executive rewards and profits, prescription drugs could be purchased at a fraction of their current covered cost.

Despite growing evidence that U.S. pharmaceutical companies are charging outrageous prices for brand-name "proprietary" drugs and making even more outrageous profits, the U.S. government has done little to curb drug costs. The government has even tried to prohibit the re-importation of drugs, at significantly lower prices, from Canada and Mexico. Why? Because the pharmaceutical industry has become the 3,000-pound gorilla of the U.S. health care industry.

---

[21] Public Citizen, "Would Lower Prescription Drug Prices Curb Drug Company R&D," April 28, 2004. Available at www.citizen.org.

[22] Marcia Angell, "The Truth About the Drug Companies," New York Review of Books, July 15, 2004, 52.

In 2003, the drug companies spent $108.6 million lobbying the federal government and hired 824 individual lobbyists.[23] Many members of Congress and other key decision-makers sit on the boards of these companies and may hold their stock as an investment. As a result, U.S. citizens have trouble getting less expensive drugs, and even Medicare (which should be the 3,000-pound gorilla in health care) is now prevented from negotiating lower drug prices for its enrollees. Yet many of these so-called "new" drugs are simply copycats of medicines already available at a much lower price, or slightly modified remakes of drugs that are no longer proprietary. The FDA does not require that a new drug be more effective than something already on the market; it must only be more effective than a placebo.

A similar accusation can be leveled at "new" technology. While much of the technology developed for medical use is critical and life-saving, many "new" devices and procedures represent only a marginal improvement over existing equipment and methods. There has also been a huge increase in disposable items for health care, all of which cost money and encourage waste. For example, when I first started practicing medicine, there was no such thing as a disposable syringe. Whether or not it is cheaper to use disposable syringes (given the time it takes to clean equipment) I am not going to argue. But today, very little is being reused, and the attitude toward disposable items encourages overuse. The rationale for this overuse may be antiseptic, but I am afraid the real reasons lie with the efforts of equipment and supply salesmen and the convenience these items offer to hospital workers. How do I know this? I have owned and managed hospitals. I know how much can be saved through the proper use of equipment and supplies.

---

[23] Public Citizen, "Drug Industry and HMOs Deployed an Army..." June 23, 2004. Available at www.citizen.org.

Other countries have done a better job of controlling the cost of new drugs and technology. In Great Britain, for example, the National Health System has established several large technological assessment centers where they independently test new procedures and new drugs to decide if they are worthwhile. While there may be additional expense involved in this, it does limit the number of products put on the market as "new and improved" that are, in fact, the same old thing. Besides, if manufacturers and drug companies know that they will be independently evaluated, they will be more hesitant about the representations they make to the public.

In the United States, we have no such controls. Medical devices and equipment, like pharmaceuticals, are sold based on hype and advertising. Each doctor and hospital in the United States insists on having the best, the newest, the most expensive tools and equipment available. A lot of the equipment could be shared among multiple providers. A mid-size city with five hospitals could probably get along with one or two imaging units, not five. But each hospital or large clinic wants its own imaging equipment. As a result, the equipment may remain idle for long periods or get used more than it needs to be. People think "it's there and available, so let's go ahead and use it." Just because the equipment is in place doesn't mean the procedure is free. Besides, because of the fee-for-service system, the owners of the equipment (whether it is an imaging device or a cardiac cath lab) will promote more expensive utilization to increase their own profits.

So what do we have? A health care system that totally fails to serve forty-five million uninsured people, and underserves millions more; health care costs that are spiraling out of control due to misuse, waste, over-utilization, new technology, pharmaceutical company greed, and an over-reliance on emergency medicine; for-profit insurance companies that exploit a system of waste and poor utilization of resources; and doctors who may be overspecialized, unavailable, and rewarded, under the fee-for-service system, for increasing the cost of health care delivery. Our citizenry, government, and industry will ultimately pay the price for all of this in neglected health and unnecessary additional costs.

The fact that our health care system is in trouble is not news to most people. Rapidly rising costs have resulted in fewer people with adequate health care coverage, and have put U.S. industries at a competitive disadvantage with other countries that have more organized and controlled health care systems. Politicians debate the problem endlessly but offer few real solutions because no one wants to get to the heart of the issue: our health care system needs major surgery, not a Band-Aid.

Medicare Reform

A variety of partial solutions have been proposed in recent years; a few have even been implemented, but to little or no effect. The most recent example is the Medicare Modernization Act of 2003. The heart of this legislation attempts to "control" the cost of prescription drugs for seniors through a strange and convoluted system of discount drug programs. Setting aside the fact that the program is unnecessarily complex, there are several major flaws in its basic design.

First, what is this discount based on? There are several price lists for the same drug used by different retail outlets. Then there is the fact that the prices are too high in the first place. So the question is: a discount off of what? Second, different discount programs each cover different drugs, leaving the patient to evaluate the cost-benefit ratio of these various plans. For the senior taking six to ten drugs a day, this may be an impossible task. Third, the program is based on an odd calculation that results in a "hole in the doughnut": below a certain level of annual expenditure, drugs are covered, and then they are not covered until you reach a higher level of expenditure. As a result, seniors who currently require moderate levels of medication may, once they reach the "hole," not be able to afford their prescriptions, which means they will get sicker and require more drugs and treatments later. Finally – and most ludicrously – the legislation prohibits the federal government from negotiating lower Medicare drug prices with the pharmaceutical companies: a transparent giveaway to the drug companies and another "home run" for the well-paid lobbyists.

From practical experience (offering various types of prescription drug coverage through our HMO over the past thirty years), I have found that discount programs do not work for the following reasons: the discount may be off an inflated retail price; prescriptions have varying dosages or number of pills; a competitor may be selling the same drug cheaper as a loss-leader; generic look-alikes are often available at lower pricing; and the patient may not be able to afford the drug, even with the discount.

A stop-loss program for the patient is the answer. This involves a maximum set price for generic prescription drugs (perhaps five dollars per prescription) and a slightly higher price for proprietary drugs (perhaps ten dollars per prescription). This kind of set price, combined with a list of drugs to be covered (formulary), can avoid wasteful duplication and the prescription of useless, unaffordable drugs. But always, there must be a published, predictable retail price for all prescriptions, and that price must be known to the patient and the doctor. The basic concept is simple: by providing drug coverage to everyone, with a stop-loss reducing waste, duplication, and misuse, we can treat more people on an ambulatory basis outside of the hospital and cut costs. Most importantly, it is not prescription drugs that cost the most; it is hospital care.

Prescription drug use in hospitals is a large, and largely hidden, problem. Strangely, drugs are fully covered by Medicare for patients in the hospital, but *not* outside of the hospital. So some Medicare patients are forced to be admitted to the hospital in order to get the drugs they need. Yet some of the most expensive drugs are used and misused in the hospital. We need proper controls in this area, particularly with regards to the most expensive and widely used drugs. Is the drug necessary? Does the doctor make use of a test dose, rather than ordering 100 pills and finding, after a few doses, that the patient can't tolerate the drug, or that it does not work? In these cases, the remaining pills are simply thrown away. In my experience, attention in this area can result in a ninety percent savings in hospital drug costs per patient stay.

We must accept the reality that without complete drug coverage, it's very difficult to treat people. They are diagnosed, but they don't take the medication. Any barrier that keeps people from getting the medication they need is detrimental to the health care system because the patients may get sicker, which will cost even more money. Any idea of limiting the amount of prescriptions per year, per individual, is self-defeating. The heaviest users are the sickest, and when the prescription supply is cut off by an arbitrary limit, they may end up in the hospital – where their care will be far more expensive but their drugs covered.

The solution to providing prescription drugs for seniors is simple: cover prescription drugs – fully – through Medicare.

This would make Medicare the largest single purchaser of pharmaceuticals in the country, which in turn would give the federal government real negotiating clout and result in a significant reduction in all drug pricing. If all forty-one million Medicare recipients could receive the appropriate medicines, we could ultimately lower the cost of providing care to seniors. The current limits on prescription drug coverage will only continue to increase medical costs in general. Medical costs are like a balloon: they include doctor care, hospital costs, and drugs; push in one side and it balloons out the other. Limit access to prescription drugs on an outpatient or ambulatory-care basis, and people will be admitted to the hospital more often (where the cost of their prescription drugs is covered).

The optimal solution to the effective use of prescription drugs is a centralized, coordinated system that controls unnecessary usage. This could be achieved through a universal data bank for all patients and prescriptions, accessed by each pharmacist through a national computer network to avoid duplication, over-dosage (resulting when patients are prescribed the same drug, with a different name, by a different doctor), and suicide. This has already been done in large HMOs.

In our staff model HMO, we employed over 100 pharmacists, several of whom worked in our central warehouse. They managed the purchasing and repackaging of all of our generic and proprietary drugs. By buying in bulk through competitive bidding, we were able to achieve a ninety percent discount on many generic drugs, which was passed on to our members. Most of these medications were machine prepackaged in preset amounts, with labeled dosage, allowing the dispensing pharmacist to increase efficiency by merely placing the patient's name and date on the package before dispensing. In our sixty pharmacies, all routine sales, packaging, and bagging were done by clerks. In addition, this pharmacy group contained several Ph.D.s in pharmacology who wrote a monthly newsletter for our medical staff outlining the effectiveness (or lack thereof) and side effects of all new drugs and treatments through an independent analysis.

The Patients' Bill of Rights

Another proposed "solution" to our health care crisis is the Patient's Bill of Rights. The "rights" this bill would ensure are: the right to have medical decisions made by a doctor, to see a medical specialist, to go to the closest emergency room, to designate a pediatrician as the primary care physician for children, to keep the same doctor throughout medical treatment, to obtain any prescription drugs the doctor prescribes, and to hold the health plan and the doctor liable for errors or untoward outcomes.

On the surface, these may sound like reasonable demands. Unfortunately, they are based on two very important – and erroneous – assumptions: that the patient is informed enough to take control of his or her own health care and that "expensive" medicine means better medicine. The problem is that the average person does not know much about health care options and treatment. A patient may want to see an orthopedic surgeon for a sprained ankle or a dermatologist for a common rash. One may insist on a pediatrician for a child's annual physical or treatment of a minor ailment, when a general practitioner is perfectly capable of performing this service. Someone else may insist on going to the emergency room for any problem, because it is more convenient than waiting for an appointment with his regular doctor. And then there are the people who go from doctor to doctor until they find a physician who agrees with their own diagnosis.

We have many competent family practitioners, nurses, and nurse practitioners in this country who are well qualified to deal with eighty percent of the common ailments most people, adults and children, experience. Patients demanding a specialist when a general practitioner or qualified family physician will do, or demanding a doctor instead of a pediatric nurse practitioner, simply drive up costs without improving the quality of care.

We also have doctors who order expensive diagnostic procedures and treatments—demanded by the patient but not really necessary—because the treatment is covered by the patient's insurance. We have doctors who write prescriptions for proprietary drugs because they were recently pitched by a drug company representative (when equally effective generic drugs are available), or who refer to a specialist when they could handle the case themselves.

Many people are under the impression that the insurance company is making health care decisions, rather than the doctor. Health insurance companies are little more than claims processors. They are not responsible for the quality, availability, or appropriateness of health care; they are responsible only for the payment. They may try to control costs by requiring the patient to see a generalist first, but it is the doctors who order the drugs, procedures, tests, referrals, and hospitalization. An insurance company may deny *payment* for care because that type of care or payment is excluded, limited, or not covered by the policy; but they cannot deny the care itself.

What we have in this country is a situation where many people purchase inexpensive, high-deductible coverage with exclusions, then want to get more expensive coverage when they need it. It is not the medical care they are being denied; it is the coverage based on the premium level of the policy they have purchased. (There is an old, bad joke that because of limitations, in order to be covered by some health and accident policies, you have to be bitten by a zebra at 4:00 PM on the freeway while you are pregnant!)

This Patients' Bill of Rights concept is based on erroneous assumptions that only serve to push the cost of health care higher. If everyone can see a medical specialist (including pediatricians) instead of a primary care physician, or go to the closest emergency room for non-emergency care; if doctors are allowed to prescribe any drug, treatment, or procedure, regardless of cost or necessity; and if health insurance companies are sued for not paying for procedures the individual's policy does not cover, we won't have "better" care. We will simply have ever-escalating health care costs without an improvement in quality.

Finally, there are a variety of ideas being tossed around by politicians – Health Care Savings Accounts, mandatory health insurance, government subsidy of catastrophic insurance, and state-funded health care coverage – that all have one thing in common: they do nothing to control the cost of health care, nor provide adequate coverage for all Americans, nor ensure the availability of care.

Health Care Savings Accounts assume that, given a tax advantage, people will voluntarily put aside money to cover health care expenses. This also assumes that everyone earns a decent income (with discretionary income to save), is logical and disciplined, and will set aside savings. If this were true, the credit card companies would be out of business. Is it realistic to think that, in a nation of individuals drowning in consumer debt and with savings levels at less than zero, these same individuals are going to set aside money for health care? Do they even have the money to set aside? These health care savings accounts are not a solution, they are wishful thinking. Even if you could convince individuals to set aside money to meet health care expenses, how much should they save? Shifting the responsibility for payment to the patient does nothing to control the cost of services or increase availability.

Legislation requiring mandatory health insurance would require everyone to purchase health insurance, with the government subsidizing those who can't afford it. The problem is no one would be mandating what the insurance companies could charge for this coverage. We have already seen this phenomenon in the COBRA (Consolidated Omnibus Reconciliation Act), which provides extended health insurance coverage after termination of employment. While insurance companies might not be able to exclude high-risk individuals under COBRA, they can certainly charge a lot more for those policies. The same problem applies to the federal government subsidizing catastrophic care: this merely shifts the payment and costs to the government without any means of controlling that cost or guaranteeing the quality and availability of care.

The idea of providing health care on a state rather than federal level has also been discussed by some legislators. Conceptually, it may be a good idea. But many metropolitan areas, such as Chicago and Cincinnati, are intersected by state lines. If health care is state-by-state, employees within the same company would have different benefits, different plans, and different coverage based on where they live. People might work in one state and live in another; which state would provide benefits? If you move, your benefits might change. Poorer states would not be able to provide the same level of benefits as larger, more affluent states. It is like trying to run the national highway system state by state; the quality and size of roads would change the minute you crossed the state line.

The basic problem is that none of the solutions proposed to date get to the heart of the problem: we need to control the cost of delivering health care while making sure everyone has access to adequate care. The only way to do this, in a fair, equitable, and effective manner, is to replace our wasteful fee-for-service system with universal coverage and the power to leverage savings through a single payer – the federal government – while offering health care providers the knowledge and incentives they need to implement that change.

Chapter 4

The Case for Universal National Health Care

The United States is the only Western industrialized country that does not guarantee adequate health care for its citizens. Basic health care – along with potable water, drivable roads, and education for our children – is something we as members of a developed-industrialized society have a right to expect. By making health care available to everyone, we can insure a healthy workforce and reduce the cost of a number of illnesses that are neglected through lack of coverage. A healthy population equates to a prosperous economy. Look at countries like Africa, where untreated diseases have depressed the economy and demoralized the population despite abundant natural resources, versus Japan with few natural resources but a healthy population.

Just about every president since Franklin D. Roosevelt has proposed some kind of national health insurance. President Harry Truman's call for a national health insurance program as part of Social Security in 1945 was countered by fierce opposition from the AMA. John F. Kennedy talked about health care, then Richard Nixon, Jimmy Carter, and Bill Clinton. They never focused on a simple, practical answer to the basic question: health care or health insurance? They didn't fully understand the issues involved in paying for and providing quality health care to everyone. Most importantly, they were intimidated and outmaneuvered by an organized opposition that created the right "Bogeyman" – national health care – and characterized it as a stepping stone to increased costs, higher taxes, and government interference with freedom of choice.

The idea that national health insurance would increase costs is an unsubstantiated myth. Data shows that we already pay more per person for health care in the United States than any other industrial nation, and get far less in return. Much of what we pay goes for insurance company marketing, advertising, profits, and provider mismanagement, resulting in unnecessary duplication and minor fraud.

Money spent on universal national health care coverage would be in place of, not in addition to, the money now being spent by public, private, and individual sources. A large portion of that money comes from state and federal government sources, which means the government is already paying for close to half the health care provided in this country – out of tax dollars. Medicare had a budget of $266.4 billion for 2004; Medicaid's budget was $280.7 billion; the Veteran's Administration health care budget was $28.4 billion.[24] That is nearly $575 billion in tax dollars for these three programs alone. Add to that the prison system, military and dependents, SCHIP (State Children's Health Insurance Program), city, county, state employee programs, government-subsidized hospitals for indigents, plus other special programs.

Assuming that providing a universal national health care program will not cost any more than we are paying now, it

---

[24] The Kaiser Commission on Medicaid and the Uninsured. The Cost of Care for the Uninsured: What Do We Spend, Who Pays, and What Would Full Coverage Add to Medical Spending? Issue Update. (The Henry J. Kaiser Family Foundation: March 2004).

follows that health care controlled by the federal government would actually *lower* the cost of health care overall for several reasons. The first is based on the insurance concept: spread the risk over a larger number of people, the sick and the healthy. If a single pool of funds is collected to cover all people – including the elderly currently covered by Medicare and the poor covered by Medicaid – the risk is spread over the entire U.S. population of nearly 300 million. Within that population, at any given moment, more people are healthy than sick. This means more people will be paying into the pool than are using services, resulting in positive financial reserves.

Secondly, by having only one entity – the federal government – paying for care, we eliminate the for-profit insurance companies as middlemen. That means we eliminate the thirty to forty percent of insurance costs that go toward marketing, administration, and profit. Paying on a prepaid capitation (per person) rate, rather than paying claims filed for each service, could virtually eliminate fraud. Finally, we can reduce the very real cost of serious illness caused by neglect or lack of access resulting in lower worker productivity, absenteeism, and more expensive treatments, including emergencies.

The majority of people in this country want some form of government-funded health care. In 1996, a Gallup Poll showed two out of three Americans favored national health insurance. I estimate that today, three out of four people would say "yes" to universal national health care, even if it meant slightly higher taxes. It is a myth that people are not willing to pay for comprehensive national health care through additional payroll taxes. Citizens of this country – like the people of most First World industrial countries – are willing to pay for services received, for a better safety net. This is, essentially, why we pay into Social Security. Shouldn't "social security" include health care? And – again – any payments for health care would *be in place of, not in addition to,* the monies individuals and employers pay now for so-called health insurance.

It is important, also, to understand that social security is not a tax: it is fundamentally a payment now for something you will need and get in the future. This is the basis of the social security retirement program. Each working person puts away money during his or her working career and then – when they retire – they receive the money back. In this same manner, if a payroll deduction is made for health care, each person will get health care paid for when it is needed. Social security is unlike taxes, which are used to pay for services you may never utilize, such as public schools (for children you don't have), highways you may never drive on, or parks you do not visit – and the military during peacetime.

A logical approach is for the federal government to take over the payment of health care for all individuals. This would eliminate health care coverage tied to employment. It would eliminate the cost of marketing and advertising health insurance (since everyone would be automatically enrolled in the government program). It could, if managed correctly, eliminate much of the fraud, waste, and duplication that currently contribute to rising health care costs.

The federal government already collects money for Social Security, which provides health care for people over the age of sixty-five. Social Security is funded by a withholding tax, paid by both the employer and the employee. A health care withholding – in place of what employers and employees now pay for private health insurance – would allow the federal government to, essentially, expand Medicare to cover everyone. When the numbers are in, I believe that any withholding for health care will be less than what employers and employees are paying today for health coverage. Payments into a universal fund would be instead of, not in addition to, current expenditures for health care.

An amazing fact is that 213 million individuals in the U.S. – more than two-thirds of the population – already have some or all of their health care coverage paid through tax dollars. This includes 21,725,000 federal employees, 21,795,300 state employees, 14,015,000 local city, county, school district, or government employees, 26,549,704 veterans, 1,444,000 military personnel (active duty and not including dependents), plus 41,086,981 Medicare and 42,400,000 Medicaid enrollees.[25] There may be some overlap of veterans who are eligible for both Medicare and veterans' benefits, and some Medicare-Medicaid and some married employees with dual coverage. But when you add to these numbers the undetermined number of employees working for counties, school districts, public universities and colleges, and other political subdivisions, it more than makes up for this overlap.

Medicare and Medicaid together cover over ninety-one million people, which is more than the population of France (sixty million) or the population of Germany (eighty million), making this group one of the largest single payer government insurance plans in the world.

The point is that between one-half to two-thirds of the population of the United States, including the military, Medicare and Medicaid, and federal, state, and public health service employees, is covered by some type of tax-supported agency or entitlement. This strengthens my argument that we are already paying enough money, either through private or

---

[25] Statistics available at www.census.gov; www.bls.gov; www.cms.gov; and www. cia.gov.

government resources, to cover everybody without additional cost or taxation.

I am not advocating "socialized" medicine. Socialized medicine means the government owns all clinics, hospitals, and medical facilities, with health care personnel working on salary for the government. Rather, I am proposing the federal government as the single payer of health care in this country. Only the federal government has the ability to fund one large risk pool through a payroll deduction. As the single payer, the federal government could negotiate hospital and physician payments even more effectively than it does now with Medicare. In addition, the federal government could negotiate prices for prescription drugs. This would make the government – rather than the pharmaceutical industry – the 3,000-pound gorilla in the health care arena.

A single pool of funds, collected and administered by the government, would expand Medicare and replace Medicaid, SCHIP, the Veteran's Administration, and private health insurance, including the health care aspect of Worker's Compensation Insurance. Also eliminated would be the tax credit – or subsidy – given to companies for providing private health insurance to their employees, an amount estimated at more than $188 billion in 2004.[26] In other words, the current, inefficient patchwork of payment systems would disappear, to be replaced by one nationwide program available to every citizen.

What We Need in a National Health Care System

Expanding Medicare to include everyone, with the federal government as the single payer, addresses the first of our three "A's":

---

[26] Kaiser Commission, "The Cost of the Uninsured." Available at www.kff.org.

affordability. Everyone would be covered, automatically, through an expanded Medicare system that offers complete health care coverage. We should, in fact, be able to offer more care because of the increased size of the risk pool and the reduction of waste, fraud, and insurance company costs and profits. Medicare, as it is funded today, is facing a serious problem: not enough money to provide health care through the present, wasteful system. By expanding Medicare to include everyone – spreading the risk over 300 million people, not forty-one million – with more and younger non-users added to the mix, the cost per person will be significantly lowered.

Medicare today covers forty-one million people, most of them over the age of sixty-five. But seniors, on average, require ten times more care than people under the age of sixty-five. This means that the current Medicare budget has to spend ten times more, per person, than an expanded Medicare. With this additional risk pool, we should be able to add prescription drugs and preventive care for all Americans without additional cost.

Perhaps the whole program can't be implemented immediately. One solution is to expand Medicare incrementally. First, we could include children and obstetric care. (Pediatricians and obstetricians are the only major doctor sector not participating in Medicare today.) Next, lower the age limit to fifty-five for Medicare recipients. Include coverage for prescription drugs, preventive care, long-term, and psychiatric care. I learned from my experience with a non-profit program (the Free Health Plan), using small clinics manned by nurse practitioners, that the largest unmet health care need is not women and children but rather the poor between age fifty-five and sixty-five with chronic disease; i.e., cardiac conditions, diabetes, neurological or degenerative illnesses.

Once this group has been integrated into the system, gradually expand Medicare to cover everyone – young and old, the employed and the unemployed. Before long, everyone will be covered under the Medicare system, and the non-functioning health "insurance" concept will collapse through the inability to spread the risk. However, a gradual process of reform will probably involve numerous fights by entrenched special interests, instead of one big battle. This incremental method also runs the risk of political "gaming" over time, crippling the program by withholding critical parts (like a "reformed" Medicare that excludes comprehensive prescription drug coverage or long-term care).

There are three elements that I believe are absolutely critical in designing a national health care system. Health care coverage *must be universal throughout all fifty states, it must be portable, and it must cover everyone, offering the same benefits to every citizen.* Universal health care, covering every citizen in the United States, means that no group, section, company, or individual can be allowed to opt out. This is because those who want to opt out (by not paying the payroll deduction) are likely to be the healthier individuals who utilize the system less, thus shifting the costs to fewer and fewer people who are sick, making it more expensive and destroying the concept of risk spread through a single-payer universal system.

The cost of health care should be part of belonging to our society, in the same way that paying taxes for schools, roads, police protection, and the military are an obligation for every citizen.

The universal aspect of paying for national health care is essential to the financial success of the program. We learned this when Medicare was introduced in 1965. Medicare consists of Part A (hospital coverage) and Part B (doctors and outpatient ambulatory services). When Medicare was first introduced, everyone was automatically covered under Part A. Part B was voluntary; Medicare recipients had to sign up for Part B and agree to have a specific amount withheld from their Social Security checks each month for this coverage.

Unfortunately, the only people who took the trouble to sign up for Part B were those who were sick. That is antithetical to the whole idea of insurance, which is to spread the risk over a large group, the healthy as well as the sick. If the healthy opt out, the costs go up for the sicker people (the users of health care) who remain in the program. When the cost or premium goes up because of subsequent greater utilization by those left, the people who are less sick drop out; the cost goes up again, and we have a death spiral for the program. (This has happened time and again with prescription drugs: the health plan with the best drug coverage gets chosen by the sickest people. This adverse selection leads to the failure of that plan.)

Social Security tried everything to get more people to sign up for Part B. They launched direct-mail campaigns to encourage people to sign up. They developed cartoon strips to encourage participation. Finally, they figured it out. They automatically enrolled everyone in Part B, maintaining choice by allowing individuals to opt out through a simple request in writing to the Secretary of Health, Education, and Welfare. If the recipient did not withdraw by letter, he or she stayed enrolled in Part B and had the deduction taken from each Social Security check automatically. The point is that the program was – technically – voluntary. But relying on the well-known factor of human inertia, this tactic worked. Very few people opted out and the cost of covering doctors' services was spread throughout the system. The lesson learned: healthy people do not pay attention to their health care coverage and do not readily or actively make changes to that coverage.

But the real lesson we learned is that you can't make payments for health care coverage voluntary. The labor unions had to learn the same lesson. They used to have cafeteria-style programs where members could choose between various benefits: health care, child care, extra vacation time, life insurance, etc. People who were healthy tended to select something other than health care. But when they had an accident or illness, they complained that they weren't covered. So, while many labor unions still offer a menu of benefit choices, health plans are no longer optional. This benefit is automatically included for all members.

Also critical is the idea that the coverage should not be job-related. Health care coverage *must be portable.* If a person loses his or her job, goes to another company, or moves to another state, that person should be able to retain the same benefits. He or she may be in the middle of treatment, expecting a baby, or have a chronic illness. This is one way in which we can be assured of a healthy population. Portability helps both employers and employees. Employers will no longer have to spend time evaluating various health plans and juggling the numbers to find a plan that fits the company's budget, or go through protracted union negotiations. Nor will they have to worry about how much health care costs will go up next year. They will know the cost of covering each person they hire and they will pay a set percentage of that person's wages into the health care fund through a payroll tax. For the employee, the portability of universal health care means the end to worrying about losing benefits by changing jobs or having to change doctors when making a career move.

This leads to the third and final basic element: *the benefits must be the same for everyone,* across the entire system. All citizens should have coverage for doctor's care, hospitalization, dental, optometry, pharmaceuticals, preventive care, and psychiatric services. We should also be looking at new ways to deal with our aging population that include but are not limited to universal in-home care, meals on wheels, elder day care or hospice in place of expensive nursing homes and hospitals, as well as alternatives to emergency room treatment, such as a network of urgent care centers, which are less expensive to staff and maintain. This means not just expanding Medicare, as it exists today, but redesigning the Medicare system to include all aspects of health care.

None of this is impossible. We are already spending enormous amounts each year on health care. The government uses tax dollars and Social Security payroll deductions to fund more than half of the health care provided in this country. *Any universal national health care program would be in place of, not in addition to,* those programs already funded by the government. Add to these funds for government programs the income from the current payroll deduction from employees and payments made by employers for private health insurance, plus deductibles and copayments paid at the time of service. Payroll deductions for universal national health insurance would replace what is currently paid for private health insurance. In fact, the cost to employers and employees should be considerably lower than it is today. A universal, single-payer health care system could eliminate copayments and deductibles, removing the biggest barriers to people seeking health care when they need it.

Health care costs will be lower overall because they will no longer include marketing, reserves, and profit for insurance companies. Expenses will be paid from a larger pool of people, most of them healthy. All of the funds in the pool, with the exception of perhaps five to ten percent for administration, will be available to pay for health care. With lower costs overall, we should be able to provide a wider range of basic health care to all citizens.

To make it truly affordable, to get the most care for the most people, and to make it accessible and available as well, the delivery of health care must be organized and managed. Only through managing the delivery and utilization of care can we eliminate the other factors that contribute to rising health care costs: fraud, duplication, waste, and marketing pressures from the big drug companies and equipment manufacturers. Why do I know this can be done? Because it already has been done through the staff model HMO and Medicare contracts with the Social Security Administration.

Chapter 5

Misconceptions, Lies, and Spin

Talking about "managed care" today is like trying to discuss communism in the McCarthy Era. People's hackles rise and they immediately become defensive. Unfortunately, managed care has – justifiably or not – been accused of poor quality, lack of service, lack of choice, roadblocks, and discontinuity of care. This is what has come of managed care under the direction of people who have nothing to do with the delivery of care: insurance companies. When you team insurance companies (who know nothing about delivering health care) with doctors (who rarely know anything about the cost of health care), you have a recipe for disaster. When I talk about managed care, I am talking about an organized system in which both the quality and the quantity of care are planned, organized, and controlled to eliminate waste and ensure that the most money is used for quality patient care. This means re-educating doctors and structuring a system that is based on patient care, not profit.

To deliver effective, quality care, we have to accept that doctors are the ones who determine the amount of care provided to patients. Doctors control the quantity and availability of care.

Hospitals don't admit patients; doctors admit patients to hospitals. Hospitals and nurses don't write the orders; doctors write the orders for procedures, medication, diagnostic tests, and length of stay. An insurance company might refuse to pay for a procedure or drug because it isn't covered under a patient's plan; but insurance companies don't order the drugs or procedures. It all starts with the doctor.

Call it management, re-orientation or re-education: doctors need to accept that proper utilization, including the organization and standardization of care, is in the best interest of the patient and the physician. Doctors must understand that just because the imaging device is there, the procedure should not be used in a cavalier manner. They need to recognize that giving the patient a variety of drugs based on the advice of the drug company representative can be counterproductive. The cardiologist orders one set of drugs, the oncologist orders another set of drugs, and when they are mixed in the stomach, the patient may be taking a whole new drug altogether.

One problem is that the practice of medicine has been skewed by the intersection of fee-for-service health care, third-party payments, and the threat of being sued for malpractice. Most doctors are still operating under a fee-for-service system, but they don't have to collect the payment for each service directly from the patient. They just send the forms on through to the insurance company or Medicare-Medicaid.

Doctors are not trained, in medical school, to "manage." This is an activity that involves careful planning, logical organization, and the development of systems and controls. Doctors are trained simply to advise patients, and are not responsible for making things happen. Yet they are expected to run their offices, recruit and train staff, manage their finances, and fulfill both staff and patients' expectations. It can happen in any organization:

poor management leads to waste, confusion, rising costs, and unhappy customers/clients/patients.

We also have to overcome the negative associations most people attach to the idea of managed care. It is a myth that "managed" care means *less* care at a lower quality. The proper utilization of health care resources means more health care is available to everyone. Under the current system, most people do *not* have coverage for prescription drugs, preventative and psychiatric treatment, or long-term care. These omissions result in an incomplete system of health care. Under a well-managed system, all these items could be covered for everyone. The increased cost of these services would be more than offset by savings through proper management of resources.

What is "quality" health care, and who determines or defines it under our current system? Is quality having a doctor who will see you the same day? Is it a doctor who is board certified in a specialty, with a number of letters after his or her name? Does quality mean seeing a doctor who will agree with your diagnosis and order whatever tests you want? Or is quality health care being able to see a doctor who is well-trained, empathetic, and conscientious? Is the doctor research-oriented or consumer-oriented? What does the average person know about selecting a doctor? How do you know where to find the appropriate physician? There are many wonderful doctors out there; there are also many poorly motivated doctors practicing with no supervision or oversight. When I was running a medical group, we had a saying: "We examine the doctor before he examines you." Good management – preferably under people educated in both medicine *and* management – can actually improve the quality of care.

It is also a myth that managed care reduces the individual's choice of doctors. Few people choose their doctor now, since insurers often specify which groups of doctors can be used. Furthermore, most people don't personally know a large number of available doctors, nor do they have the knowledge to evaluate a doctor's qualifications. A well-run managed care system can actually offer a better, more educated choice by providing information to the patient about each provider. We used to keep a loose-leaf binder at the front desk of each clinic with the photos and résumés of forty or forty-five internists for patients to choose from. Where can the average person access that kind of information – on forty different internists – in private practice? At best, the IPA or PPO – which are not really HMOs – may provide a list with names and addresses, but that's it.

In addition to fearing a lack of "choice," people also equate managed care with rationed care. This is a fallacy. For one thing, if a health plan does not give the proper amount of care, they risk losing the patient as a customer or even losing the whole employer group. Lack of availability or poor quality care will often result in more expensive hospital or intensive care. Avoidance of this is the real financial incentive for providing early treatment and keeping the patient healthy. Under managed care, it only makes sense to give each person the appropriate amount of care ("appropriate" being the key term here).

Consumers, as well as doctors, need to be re-educated in how they look at health care delivery. They need to understand the role of the individual doctor as a caregiver, not a businessperson. They need to see that health care, like much else in life, is a system with limited resources. This means that we need to combine the skills of the caregiver with the practical expertise of a manager to provide the best possible level of care to the most people.

Lessons Learned from Managed Care

This country has had one successful form of managed care: the staff model Health Maintenance Organization. In the staff model, everyone works on salary, in clinics owned and managed by the HMO. The HMO enrolls patients on a capitation basis, charging so much per person, per month in exchange for providing all health care services.

Unfortunately, the staff model HMO – with the exception of Kaiser's organization, the military, and a few others – has not survived. It worked, and it worked well when properly managed and financed, but it was ultimately undercut by pressure from special interests and their spin artists, investors desiring to make a profit, doctors poorly trained in management, and negative press.

In fact, in the 1970s, the federal government sponsored a whole network of staff model HMOs. They recognized the savings potential of this form of delivery system. Unfortunately, most of these HMOs failed for the usual reasons: they were under-financed and under-managed by doctors and academics. What we need today is not to resurrect the staff model HMO but to design a new form of organized delivery system. Nevertheless, there are lessons learned from the staff-model HMO that can be applied to planning for a new national health care delivery system.

Lesson number one: *Paying a capitation rate – so much per person, per month—to an organization that directly provides health care services, can cut health care delivery costs by twenty-five percent to fifty percent.* How do I know this? My organization (FHP, a staff model HMO), with our first capitated project for Medi-Cal/Medicaid, saved twenty-five percent on costs, and delivered care that was as good as, or better than, fee-for-service. This was according to a report by the State of California legislative analyst, examining the Family Health Program (FHP) MediCal Demonstration Project, a Department of Health Care Services contract to provide comprehensive services through capitated prepayment. The analysis found that:

> FHP charges were 19 percent lower for OAS (old age and survivors) patients and 27 percent lower for AFDC (aid to families and dependent children) patients than in neighboring Los Angeles….We think that FHP is a fiscally sound program which could be used as a model for small and medium sized groups designed to practice this type of medicine. We are not qualified to comment on the quality of care under FHP but are not aware of any major problems as of this writing.[27]

These findings, by an unbiased third party, appear to verify the concept that a prepaid capitated staff model HMO can provide managed care of equal quality for a significant savings as opposed to the usual fee-for-service system. (Later on, as FHP grew and experienced more economies of scale, and the fee-for-service costs became higher, we were able to save 50% on hospital bed days alone with our 1985 Medicare contract.)

The managed care organization provides the service and is responsible for controlling over-utilization (duplication of tests and services, over-prescription of expensive drugs, or excessive hospital utilization) and over-billing. This health care service provider is, at the same time, responsible for the quality of care. It is in their best interest to keep people well and out

---

[27] "Report of the Legislative Analyst to the Joint Legislative Budget Committee," Analysis of the Budget Bill of the State of California for the Fiscal Year July 1, 1971 to June 30, 1972 (Sacramento, CA: California Legislature, 1971 Regular Session), 14-16.

of the hospital. Under this system, the provider does not get paid more for putting the patient in the hospital and/or doing marginal procedures. If they do not provide quality service, that patient will get sicker and require more care, costing the provider organization more. With capitation payments, there are no claims to file, as we have under the current insurance system. This cuts down on excessive billing as well as the administrative expense of paying claims.

The case for paying a capitation rate has been proven again and again as the government has attempted to control the cost of Medicare, but capitation must work hand-in-hand with managed care. In the late 1960s, I was asked to be a consultant for Social Security (SSA) in Baltimore in order to devise a prepaid capitated system for compensating physicians for Medicare services. Along with SSA executives and other consultants, we designed a plan in Baltimore that would do just that by emphasizing ambulatory care rather than hospitalization. Unfortunately, this plan was a failure. The harder the doctors tried to do as much as possible on an ambulatory basis, the more work they had to do for the same payment per head. The problem was that while more care on an ambulatory basis resulted in less expensive hospitalization, benefiting the whole system financially, the doctors received little financial reward for their efforts. This was corrected in the mid 1980s, when Social Security began awarding contracts to doctor groups and other HMOs to provide and pay for ambulatory as well as hospital service. This allowed these organizations to benefit financially from their efforts to do more on an ambulatory basis and decrease the high cost of hospital utilization. In these programs, the hospital utilization was cut in half with no discernable effects on the quality of care. An added benefit was that the less time people spent in the hospital, the better off they were.

The first Medicare capitated prepaid contracts were developed in the mid-1980s by the Social Security Administration, with total medical and hospital benefits being supplied and paid for by the group practice prepayment organization. The government paid these organizations, on contract, a set amount per month per individual as a prepaid monthly capitation rate equal to ninety percent of what they paid the fee-for-service sector for fewer services. This was actually closer to seventy percent, since they were paying on a trailing three-year average instead of a projected next-year's average, which was when the service would be rendered. Nevertheless, medical groups were able to realize a savings in the hospital sector by providing more ambulatory care services and more careful hospital utilization. The hospital utilization under the prepaid health care plans was approximately one half of what it was in the fee-for-service sector: 1,500 hospital bed days per 1,000 individuals covered per year, rather than 3,000 hospital bed days per 1,000 individuals covered per year. This savings produced additional income to the medical groups, which they could spend on providing more ambulatory care and additional benefits, while eliminating deductibles and copayments.

Before I established my first Medicare contract with the federal government in 1984, I visited several existing Medicare prepaid group practice pilot projects. Some of them were succeeding and some of them were failing. The reasons for success or failure became obvious and provided lessons for the future. Those who tiptoed into taking Medicare on a capitation rate by enrolling a small number of people, or those who charged a premium, failed. The ones who succeeded charged no premium and made the commitment to sign up a large number of Medicare patients for a set rate, which spread the risk and allowed them to offer a full range of services above and beyond what was required by the Medicare contract. They were also willing to spend time and money on education, marketing, and sales to acquire a significant enrollment quickly. Charging a premium and covering a smaller number of individuals guaranteed the enrollment of only the sick: a path to failure.

Our program of extending coverage beyond Medicare, at no premium, in our first contract in Long Beach was so popular we enrolled 10,000 Medicare people in six weeks. We covered doctor care, hospitalization, prescription drugs, psychiatric care, and preventive care – with no premium, no deductible, and no copayment. Our two specially designed senior centers were open twelve hours a day, seven days a week, to serve our Medicare patients. In other words, we were able to make health care affordable, available, and accessible. One flat monthly rate paid for by an entity other than the individual recipient was, in this case, an important concept in maintaining individual enrollment. Health care must be paid for by an organization (e.g. an employer or the government) rather than the individual, because many individuals do not include health care in their budget.

I believed we could offer the full range of services because we could control the utilization of those services. By my calculation, there was at least fifty percent waste and erroneous billing in the federal government fee-for-service Medicare sector overall. The biggest cost was in hospital care due to over-utilization. We could offer a full-service health care program without charging a monthly premium (additional payment by the individual), copayment or deductible, and still cover our marketing, reserve requirements, development costs, and a reasonable net out-of-hospital savings on better utilization control alone.

The plan that I negotiated with Social Security, which was the first prepaid health care contract on the West Coast, established the policy for subsequent Medicare contracts. In this plan, we were able to accept payment at ninety percent of the amount paid to the fee-for-service sector for Medicare services and eliminate the copayment on ambulatory care plus the deductible for each hospitalization. We were also able to add prescription drugs on a formulary basis. Preventive care, such as immunizations, physical examinations, counseling and psychiatric care, and eye examinations and glasses were added as well. We did all this for – surprise – no premium.

The beauty of this program was the "no premium." This meant that the healthy, in addition to the sick, would join the program. My investigation of the pilot projects that had preceded our program helped me to develop valid conclusions to create a successful, capitated program for Medicare. The conditions for success were as follows:

1. There must be no premium. If a premium is charged, only sick people join the health plan, healthy people will not, and the program is doomed from its inception. This is akin to writing fire insurance only on houses that are on fire.

2. The total payment for health care must be made by a third party.

3. At least 10,000 people must be enrolled quickly, to establish a large enough risk pool; this means allocating and budgeting resources for marketing.

4. The program has to cover prescription drugs for little or no payment. It is an exercise in futility to treat people who are unable to purchase the drugs that are prescribed.

5. Hospitalization has to be controlled; elective services have to have prior authorization and second opinions to make sure that they are necessary. Hospitalization itself has to be organized so that people are released from the acute hospital to sub-acute hospitals and then to home care (with visiting nurses) on a planned basis, followed by outpatient rehabilitation services.

Which brings me to lesson number two: *Copayments and deductibles place a barrier between the doctor and the patient.* This is what preventive care is all about: removing the barrier between the doctor and the patient with early treatment, health evaluations, immunizations, and wellness programs. It is a myth that if you remove the copayment, you will be inundated by hypochondriacs. The reality is that people are reluctant to go to the doctor because it takes time, is inconvenient and sometimes demeaning, and they may receive bad news. If copayments are added to these psychological barriers, people will postpone seeing a doctor until they absolutely have to – in other words, when they are very sick and need a lot of care.

In reality, making preventive care effective takes a lot of education. Even with annual physicals fully covered on all of our plans, the best we could ever do was twenty-five percent utilization. When we enrolled new Medicare patients, we would send a van out to pick them up and bring them in for an evaluation. If they had a chronic disease, like diabetes, we wanted them under treatment right away. We did not want to wait until they got worse or needed hospitalization.

Preventive care simply does not work on a fee-for-service basis. The first insurance company I chartered – to provide companion dual-choice health and accident insurance as an alternative to an HMO – was the HMO Life Insurance Company. This was the first health insurance company in California to require prior authorization for elective hospitalization. The program was very successful because the fee-for-service doctors could not, or would not, write-up requests for elective hospitalization that were questionable, and our hospital utilization rate dropped. These savings in hospital costs provided a financial basis that we thought would allow us to provide preventive care such as immunizations and annual health evaluations, eventually controlling costs even more. However, many of the fee-for-service doctors soon figured out a way to make a profit from this preventive service: they gamed the system so that anybody who walked into a doctor's office was immediately billed for a complete physical and given a series of immunizations, whether they needed it or not. Our insurance company quickly went from a profit position to a loss position. This company was eventually converted into a company that provided an alternative coverage to the HMO by fee-for-service doctors, with a deductible and copayment to the HMO, at the same price as the HMO, with life insurance over the top. (The lesson learned: The inability to control some independent fee-for-service community doctors killed off this concept of preventive care.)

This example indicates why, under the fee-for-service concept, expanding coverage and containing costs does not work as it does under the managed care capitated system. Preventive care can only be provided through an Organized Provider System (OPS), where the doctors and providers are responsible for the patient's total care for a flat monthly sum and have no incentive to exploit the system.

The accessibility of prescription drugs is another major component of preventive care. We realized that charging a large copayment for prescription drugs created a barrier to patients getting the needed medications, so we kept the copayment low (between five and ten dollars), providing a stop-loss for the recipient. In other words, the patient always knew the maximum they would have to pay. We were able to do this because we were careful about what drugs were available in our formulary (as determined by our pharmacy department, not drug company representatives) and we used about eighty percent generic, prepackaged drugs. In addition, our pharmacies were computerized with a central list of patient medications. For efficiency and cost control, the pharmacies were systemized, so all of the bagging, cash, and counter work were done by pharmacy aides, leaving the pharmacist time to consult with patients or verify dispensing.

Lesson number three: *The seamless, vertical integration of services is essential in providing better quality health care at a lower cost.* Everything has to be managed and integrated, from the ambulance service to hospitals, doctors, and pharmacy services. How can you effectively deliver health care if you only manage a piece of it?

We did this with Medicare. When people enrolled in our program, they gave up their Medicare cards in exchange for our enrollment cards, assuring more benefits with no copayment or deductible. We took responsibility for providing all their care, including pharmaceutical. When the patient filled a

---

[31] Kaiser Family Foundation, "Public Cites Health Care as Second Most Important Problem for Government to Address," August 29, 2005. Posted at www.kff.org.

prescription at one of our pharmacies, the pharmacist could go into the computer and see if that patient just filled another prescription for that drug. Or she could see that he shouldn't take that drug because it could have a harmful interaction with something else he was taking, as listed in our data bank. The patient wouldn't end up with several bottles of drugs he didn't or couldn't use. When a patient was admitted to one of our hospitals, the doctor had immediate access to a complete medical history involving every provider and enrollee within the system – treatments, medications, diagnoses, tests, and procedures.

Another advantage of integrating services was that our doctors worked together as a team, rather than as individuals in their own offices. Working in a team meant the doctors could pool their knowledge for proper treatment and were better positioned to catch any mistakes or oversights. There's an old Chinese saying: "When many eyes are watching, few bad things happen." More doctors sharing information and expensive equipment meant better care at a lower cost. Integrating the medical, hospital, and pharmaceutical services ensured continuity of care for our patients.

Lesson number four: *There are better – and more cost-effective – alternatives to hospitalization and emergency care.* A significant percentage of people who go to emergency rooms need urgent care, not emergency services. Some hospitals end up closing their emergency rooms because they were overwhelmed with patients seeking routine ambulatory care who have no means of paying for services. The closure of Drew-King Center in the Watts-Compton area of Los Angeles will force many poor people into surrounding hospital emergency rooms, where they will be seen for initial treatment and referral, creating an overwhelming situation for these already overworked hospitals. (Eventually, those hospitals should welcome universal health care, which will guarantee payment for all services rendered.)

The hospital sector is poorly controlled in the United States. This enormous cost center consists of a conglomeration of community hospitals, public hospitals (county, city, medical school, military, and prison), religious order hospitals, and private non-profit and for-profit hospitals (some proprietary and some public with shareholders). Many of these hospitals are struggling to stay afloat in an environment that is both competitive and ruinously expensive.

There are numerous ways that hospitals can control costs; I could write a book about that alone. Hospitals will probably respond that it is the doctors who order the procedures, so the doctors are responsible for cost overruns. The answer to that is for hospitals to educate their medical staff. We did it! Hospitals can and should compete on a consumer service and comfort level, not only in acquiring new equipment and expensive add-ons. Unfortunately, many hospitals encourage doctors to overuse their underused facilities, such as cardiac surgery and imaging departments, in the belief that this is the only way to recoup the cost of their investment in equipment and facilities. They make these investments in the belief that doctors will not use their facilities otherwise. It is a vicious circle that leads to over-utilization of hospitalization and expensive procedures, resulting in spiraling health care costs.

The difference in hospital utilization rates between an uncontrolled health and accident insurance plan and an organized system is spectacular. When I retired from FHP in the late 1990s, our hospital utilization rate was about 300 bed days per thousand individuals per year. The Blue Cross rate was 600 per thousand individuals covered per year. Our average all-in cost per day for an acute hospital was $1,400 a day compared to the fee-for-service rate of $1,600 per day, even though our patients were only admitted to the hospital for severe illness. This was due to our extensive outpatient treatment system. The insurance companies realized the profitability of contracting for Medicare under this system but could not figure out how to make it work. They rapidly bought up the small start-up Medicare-contracting HMOs and incorporated them into their client base. Then they began complaining about the low rates paid by Medicare, because the insurance companies were unable to control the utilization as originally conceived and accomplished by the HMOs they had acquired. This – falsely – gave the whole HMO concept a bad reputation.

As 1985 became 1995 and 2005, the population originally enrolled in Medicare under the group practice prepayment concept began aging. They were no longer in their late sixties but in their eighties, with many more serious illnesses. The more that was done for the octogenarians, the longer they lived, and the more costly their care became. Without the influx of active marketing for new, younger enrollees or the allocation of new enrollees to the program, the costs rose rapidly. With the proliferation of new, expensive diagnostic and treatment procedures, the cost increased further. This could have been controlled by doctor groups if they wanted to do so. Since the insurance companies are not known for their long-range thinking, they did not care that by about 2010, the seventy-five million baby boomers in their sixties born after World War II would begin to edge into the Medicare system, which would have the effect of decreasing overall utilization by lowering the average Medicare age. Inclusion of this new, larger, and younger Medicare group will be added to what remains of the forty million-plus original Medicare recipients. With a lower average age and lower overall utilization of this new, larger group, Medicare prepayment contracts should indeed be profitable.

Looking beyond the present, we developed a long-term program that further decreased hospital costs: the "sub-acute" hospital. Realizing that acute (full-service) hospitals were focusing more and more on intensive care, with prices to match, we developed the sub-acute hospitals as something midway between an acute hospital and a skilled-nursing facility. As a pilot project in California, we purchased two skilled-nursing hospitals, gutted and refurnished them, and increased the nursing staff. The result was quiet, comfortable garden hospitals without X-ray labs or expensive surgery facilities. Patients in the acute hospitals who were stabilized after two or three days were transferred to these sub-acute hospitals. The formula was simple: a $100 ambulance transfer changed a $1,400-a-day acute hospital cost to a $215-a-day sub-acute hospital cost and produced a significant savings with better service and comfort for the patient. Upon release from these sub-acute hospitals, the patient's progress was followed by our home nursing staff. This system of combining acute hospital care with sub-acute hospital and home nursing care requires volume to survive financially, but it has been proven to be efficient and effective.

In fixing the current system of health care delivery to control excessive rising costs and ineffective, wasteful non-systems, a whole group of new and innovative programs like these must be developed. There are reasons behind reasons for various non-functioning health care sectors. One example is the overcrowding of emergency rooms (ERs) in the inner cities. The unemployed, the working poor, and the uninformed and uneducated seek their health care in ERs, mostly county hospitals, and sometimes medical schools and private hospitals. These people may or may not be eligible under Medicaid, and they may or may not know it. Basically, they have little concept of obtaining care through a private doctor; their first thought is to go to the emergency room.

There are other reasons some people turn to the ER for routine care. They may not have transportation available during the day, or they may work at low-paying jobs that do not allow for paid time off to visit a doctor (e.g., hotel maids and construction workers), or there may be no babysitter, or they may simply have bigger problems to deal with. When someone in this situation gets sick, there is no option but to go to the ER.

One solution to the overuse of ERs is small neighborhood clinics staffed by nurse practitioners (with several clinics supervised by one doctor) open evenings until 8:00 PM and all day Saturday and Sunday. These health clinics – or stations – could provide routine health care as well as health and community education such as "How to Know When You Are Sick" and "Where to Go for Help."

We have done these types of programs successfully. On the Island of Yap, an isolated community in the middle of the Pacific, we ran a pilot project using thirty ten-foot-by-ten-foot health care centers, each staffed by a trained health aide. At these centers, we immunized ninety-eight percent of the population of 7,000, provided basic health services, plus family planning and minor care, and reduced the occupancy of their fifty-bed hospital from 100 percent to ten percent. This was accomplished through simple preventive care that ended infantile diarrhea and indigenous diseases such as cholera, malaria, or measles, and reduced infant and preschool mortality and unplanned pregnancies.

In the Free Health Plan in Orange County, California, we duplicated the Outer Island isolated rural delivery system with five small, inner-city installations, each manned by a nurse practitioner and an assistant, and all five supervised by one doctor qualified in family practice. This system of small clinics was both effective and low-cost. It was here we were able to document an interesting observation: the most care is needed for people between the ages of fifty-five and sixty-five with chronic, treatable illness, not children or pregnant mothers.

Yes, there are multiple community clinics here and there in many urban areas. But some are open only a few hours a week, and many are limited to offering special services such as family planning, dental, or counseling services. The point is that there are few planned community networks designed to cover an entire city area *and* offering basic primary health care on an accessible, available basis. We certainly don't have a similar program to cover the whole United States.

In our hospitals, we took the pressure off the ER by opening Urgent Care Centers next door to the ER. Emergency room service is usually defined as life-threatening conditions such as trauma, an inability to breathe, intense pain, unconsciousness, and a few other definitive conditions. Urgent care is about something that needs to be taken care of today (usually when no doctors' offices are open) but is not necessarily life-threatening.

Our Urgent Care Centers were open evenings and weekends. Patients utilized the Urgent Care Center for a variety of reasons: they did not want to take time off from work to see the doctor; they did not want to wait for an appointment; their condition suddenly got worse; or the one family car was only available in the evening. In urgent care, there are no appointments. Doctors see patients on a first-come, first-served basis, resulting in varied waiting time, since the attending doctor never knows what will be seen next – a hangnail or a heart condition.

The alternatives to utilizing expensive hospital care are numerous and varied. In Utah, our centers along the Wasatch Front (Ogden, Salt Lake City, and Provo) served over one half of the (mostly Mormon) Utah population. This was a homogeneous population with families of five to seven children each. To meet the needs of this specific population, we developed outpatient obstetrical delivery centers (birthing centers) with an obstetrics unit identical to the hospital's obstetric facilities. It was near the hospital, with immediate ambulance service in case of complications. These centers were only for women who had delivered before with no complications. Most of the time, the father was in attendance. Deliveries were done by trained midwives, backed by an attending obstetrician on site.

After twenty-four hours, provided there were no problems, we would discharge the mother and baby. Then a nursing service visited the mother and infant at home each day, to check on their condition and teach the mother proper newborn care. This type of service offered a practical advantage in orienting the mother to early infant care at home, a benefit not usually available in the hospital setting. As a special twist, instead of the usual insurance company practice of charging a copayment for each delivery, we gave the mother a set amount of money to hire a mother's helper. This was a very popular program. It provided better care for both mother and baby and precluded a three-day hospital stay, resulting in a $6,000 savings in an area of high utilization. It also illustrates that in health care, one size does not fit all. Because of cultural differences, innovative and creative alternatives may be appropriate and cost-effective.

Lesson number five: *"Managed" care requires people trained as managers.* This may mean professional managers with a specialization in health care delivery, or it may mean doctors or other health care professionals who have received training as managers. There is a significant difference between a medical provider (usually a doctor) and a manager. Doctors are advisors. They are not responsible for making anyone do anything; they only recommend. Managers, on the other hand, must make things happen. They must conceive a plan, identify problems, and set about developing a solution and achieving a result. Many times, a doer is misplaced as an advisor and an advisor is misplaced as a doer. This can happen in any field.

If you think about it, doctors do not really have a long-term career path; they finish medical school, complete an internship and/or residency, and then proceed to do the same thing for the next forty or fifty years. There are many doctors who, after ten or fifteen years of practice, welcome the chance to do something different. To help some of these doctors expand their horizons, and knowing that there was a dearth of trained, qualified doctor-managers in the country, I set about creating a program in the 1970s that was team-taught by our HMO and the University of California, Irvine, School of Management. We required that all attendees were currently serving in some managerial or supervisory position. For instance, they could be a department chair, a clinic medical director, a chief pharmacist, or a dental director.

This two-semester course was taught at the university one weekend a month (Friday through Sunday, with Thursday and Monday for travel from our outlying regions). The university provided the faculty, and we team-taught. For instance, their professor of finance and our CFO taught the finance section together. The same system was used for classes in marketing, operations, human factors, and other areas. It was a sixteen-week course with tracks for the various management concepts. The students graded the professors, and as we moved along, we substituted some of the university faculty for outside consultants. (These students were mature doctors with advanced degrees who would not tolerate poor performance by professors that might be accepted by the average student simply seeking a grade.)

Some of the doctors were suited to management training and became excellent managers; others, after taking the course, preferred to continue in the clinical setting. At the very least, after finishing the course, the physicians became familiar with the problems of management and how to go about finding solutions. This created a tremendous morale boost in the medical team because it helped eliminate the "us versus them" (doctors versus management) view traditionally held by some medical practitioners. Incidentally, I never had a doctor who moved into full-time management voluntarily want to return to clinical medicine.

Through this system, I believe we trained over half the medical directors in the United States in the 1980s. Our experience with the management training program for doctors is the basis for my suggestion that the educational system for doctors be divided into three tracks. The first would be the clinical track for individuals who have the personality to become successful caregivers and enjoy working directly with patients, solving diagnostic problems, and being advisors. The second is for those who wish to become researchers, physicians who are more scientifically oriented and have less empathy for interacting with people. (Unfortunately, today we have some clinicians who are better suited to be techno-scientists than caregivers.) The third track would be for individuals who are action-oriented, strategic thinkers, who want to get into management and make things happen.

We could end up with higher-quality health care by providing three tracks in medical schools for these various personality types. It is inappropriate to think that everybody who goes to medical school in their early twenties knows what they want to do for the rest of their lives *and* has the personality to be a clinician. That just doesn't happen. Recognizing that different personality types are suited to different roles in health care will allow us to make the best use of our medical resources. If a doctor works in one track for ten years then decides to change, or becomes better suited to a different track, that doctor can retrain and move to an alternate sector.

Effective managed care also requires more people well-trained in *all* aspects of health care. The apparent shortage of medical personnel in the U.S. – doctors, nurses, and medical technicians of various types – is due to inadequate planning and a lack of opportunity for those people who are intelligent and qualified to become doctors. Many people face significant economic barriers to getting the training they desire and need.

Our experience in solving the nursing shortage is illustrative. When we were about to open our first hospital, I asked my hospital management team where they were going to get their nursing staff. Their answer was that they would simply pay ten percent more and steal the nurses from the other hospitals. I let them know this was an unacceptable answer; the other hospitals would counter by offering ten percent more than we were paying and attempt to build it into their fee schedule. So we developed a program to solve the problem of a nursing "shortage."

The first thing we did was poll our licensed vocational nurses (who were not RNs but rather assisted the nurses) to find out how many of them would like to become registered nurses. Then we administered a series of intelligence and personality tests to find out who would be appropriate. When we identified the people who both wanted to become RNs and had the intellectual and personal ability to do so, we enrolled them in training, paid for their tuition and books, and paid them a salary while they were in training.

Why did we pay them a salary? Because even with the cost of tuition and books covered, many of them had dependents and could not forgo income to advance their careers. In return for this salary, they worked for us for about three hours a day while they were in school and agreed to work for our hospital at the regular pay level for two years after graduation. The vast majority of these people stayed with us for years because they appreciated the opportunity.

Later on, we established a similar program for RNs who wished to become intensive care nurses. This involved a period of time in training at the medical school, studying the intricacies of working in the intensive care ward. Again, we paid their tuition, books, and salary while they took courses at the university medical school. We also established low-cost child care centers for employees' children near the hospitals. As a result, we always had a good supply of intensive care nurses.

Our long-range plan was to recruit people from low-income areas who wanted to get into the nursing profession to be nursing assistants. From there, we planned to pay for their training and salary to become licensed vocational nurses, then we would move the more qualified people to the RN training and then from there to intensive care nursing through the same system.

This shows that there is a creative solution for every problem. The solution here was to provide the necessary education and adequate compensation while medical providers were in training. There is nothing new about this idea. In World War II, the federal government paid for most doctors' medical school training, gave them a salary, tuition, and books, and even gave them clothes (albeit khaki or navy blue) while they went to medical school. Today, the military continues to train physicians while providing them officers' compensation and benefits.

The sixth and final lesson we can learn from managed care is that *everyone must have the same benefits.* If you offer a varied menu of health care options to people, effective management and utilization go out the window. People will choose only what they think they may need, and expect to pay less if they choose fewer options. This means people will forgo some services and may not have the care they need, when they need it.

I made this mistake early on when I added elective obstetric care to our individual programs for an extra two dollars per month, per family. We collected $18 over nine months and then the family dropped the obstetric care but kept the other benefits. That didn't work. If you provide obstetric care, or any other benefit, you have to offer it to everybody. The rate paid by people who are *not* pregnant helps to pay for pregnancies. The rate paid for people not requiring surgery pays for the people who do. The only way to make a national health care program work is to offer everyone the same benefits and pay the same set amount for everyone. This payment may be modified for cost differences in different markets or geographic areas, but the payment must provide the same benefits for everyone, regardless of where they live or work.

The term "managed care," as it is used now, represents nothing more than a marketing effort by insurance companies posing as HMOs. True managed care involves a vertical integration of services, with payments made directly to the service providers who are then responsible for utilization and quality. It means removing the barriers between doctors and patients by eliminating copayments and deductibles, and educating physicians to coordinate and manage their time and the utilization of resources better. It means developing more efficient and cost-effective means of making the same level of health care available to all Americans.

Chapter 6

Why Change is Difficult and What to Do About It

Every attempt at reforming health care in this country has been met with resistance from organized medicine, which includes the American Medical Association, state medical associations and specialty groups, the insurance and hospital associations, the pharmaceutical industry, and all the lobbyists for these groups. Why? Because for national single-payer health care to work, they will have to change the way they do business. Remember the commercial that aired in the 1990s, when Hillary Clinton tried to develop a national health plan? It showed two people sitting at the breakfast table, worrying that a national plan would take away their "choice" and lead to poor quality care. This was paid for by the HIAA (Health Insurance Association of America) and was nothing more than "spin" designed to confuse the issue.

Opponents to single-payer health care can't offer *real* reasons why it would be bad for the American public, so they attempt to confuse that public by playing on imagined fears to block any true change. If you can't defeat them, confuse them. The only real fear is on the part of these opponents to single-payer national health care. If the federal government is paying for all health care in this country, the doctors, the insurers, and the pharmaceutical companies will be in bed with a 3,000 pound gorilla that can set limits on what they charge for their products and services, can establish a truly competitive system, and can organize the current inefficient, wasteful mess.

When I first started thinking about universal coverage funded by a single payer, it seemed that everyone *should* be for it. Employers should support it because they would no longer face the annual chore of shopping for health plan coverage, union negotiations, and raises in health care premiums. Doctors should be for it because they would see an increase in paid-for patients – not a bad deal. They could stop worrying about the confusing plethora of insurance forms and varied benefits, and would no longer have to file mountains of claims.

Consumers should be for it, because they would have access to health care, no matter where they live or who they work for. Even suppliers to the health care industry – drug companies and equipment manufacturers – should be for it (even though they may have smaller profit margins) because their market will be larger; more people would have access to health care. There really shouldn't be anybody against it except those profiting from the current system. The established medical industry (health insurers, for-profit hospitals, drug companies, and unenlightened doctors) has vehemently opposed universal national health care. In fact, the roadblocks to national universal health care can be divided into three groups: insurers, providers, and suppliers. These roadblocks are enabled by a fourth group: policy makers.

Insurers

Insurance companies are *not* health care providers. Their business is insuring against risk (the one-time possible event), not an inevitable, recurring need (health care). Their mission is defined by revenue and the next quarter's financial report. They have profited hugely by getting into the non-discretionary health "insurance" field. If costs go up, they just raise their premiums. This profit would decline sharply if the federal government were in a position to set limits on how much is paid for the delivery of health care and to demand competitive practices.

Today, health and accident insurance simply does not work as a cost effective means of delivering health care. Insurance companies don't control cost, quality, or accessibility; these are all determined by doctors. The use of insurance companies as a third-party payee simply increases health care costs by adding at least thirty percent in marketing, administration, and profit (not including the cost of fraudulent claims). And that profit is what makes insurance companies determined to stay in the health care field. That's why they will pay for the lobbyists, contribute to the negative advertising designed to confuse voters, and block any rational form of national health care.

Insurance companies could, conceivably, play a role in a universal national health care system by providing "add-on" benefits or getting involved with the "additional choice" second tier I mentioned earlier. Or they could handle the administration of claims for the federal government, as they do now for Medicare. The point is that insurance companies can remake themselves as something else. They are a part of the financial services industry, where the majority of profits come from providing financing, not underwriting. These companies entered the health insurance business only fifty or so years ago, so they can once again change the role they play.

Providers

Organized medicine has consistently opposed any plan that will take away the "patient's right to choose," assuming that most

Americans know how to select a doctor or hospital and have a wide selection to choose from. It is hard to understand the logic behind this form of opposition. In the first place, it is a myth that most people consistently see one particular doctor. Most people are reasonably healthy and, if they need health care, they will probably choose the doctor who is most convenient in terms of location, has been selected by their insurer, or has been recommended by a friend or relative. "Choice" is not the primary factor. Even if it were, few people know how to evaluate a physician's qualifications.

There is an additional source of "lack of choice" within the current system: the tendency of many doctors to close their practices to new patients. It is hard to understand this regressive type of thinking, since in the very nature of medicine, a doctor's practice decreases as patients die or leave the area. As the patient base decreases in size, only way a doctor can maintain income levels without taking in new patients is by increasing the services and the cost of services to the current patient base. (This could be construed as anti-social behavior since some part of every doctor's education is paid by public tax dollars. Rather than restricting the practice or making it difficult for patients to get in, doctors have a social obligation to hire and train associates to share the burden of the practice and expand it to include all citizens in need of care.) What we have is a decrease in available doctor services, even as the number of doctors remains constant. This is another reason to increase the number of doctors trained in the U.S.

Well-managed national health care would in fact give people more – not less – choice because they will be able to afford the care they need, regardless of the doctor. There's no point in being able to choose a physician if a person lacks the ability to pay for that physician's services. A well-managed national health care plan will also bring an end to duplication and excess utilization. This is what the AMA really fears: a federal government program that can set limits on the amount and pricing of services.

In the 1960s, I published a paper with the UCLA School of Public Health providing a case study illustrating that seventy percent of people enrolled in a prepaid health plan did not care what doctor they went to, as long as he or she seemed qualified.[28] Furthermore, when given the opportunity to choose between a more expensive insurance plan with unlimited choice of doctors or a prepaid health plan with more coverage and a more limited group of doctors, they overwhelmingly chose better coverage over choice of doctor.

That first case study was based on the break-up of an early group practice in which the individual's choice was between the prepaid medical group (most of the original doctors had left the group) and a more expensive insurance coverage with unlimited choice. Most of the consumers gave up their doctors and kept the prepaid plan, proving that the coverage is more important than the doctor.

A later case study, in 1986, analyzed a situation in which patients were given the choice of either staying with a known hospital in the community on a more limited insurance program, or joining a prepaid group plan that offered another hospital in another community with more benefits and a better premium rate. Again, seventy percent chose to change hospitals and keep their more inclusive, less expensive plan. This belies the myth that most people want or need

---

[28] Shirley Rich, Robert Gumbiner, M.D. and Milton I. Roemer, M.D., "The Doctor or the Plan: A Test of Family Prioirties," *Inquiry* Vol. 6, no. 2 (1968), 59-61.

to "choose" their doctor or hospital.[29] (For more on these studies, see Appendix A.)

Organized medicine is consistently opposed to anything that threatens the sanctity of the independent, fee-for-service physician, yet few people coming out of medical school today will "hang up a shingle" and start an individual, private practice. Less than twenty-five percent of all doctors working in the United States today operate as solo practitioners. The solo practitioner, working alone and on call twenty-four hours a day, seven days a week, is becoming an anachronism, as should the idea that this doctor deserves a high level of income in exchange for taking on all the risk and working around the clock.

Today, the majority of doctors work in groups in which they "share call" and/or refer "after-hours patients" to organized emergency rooms or urgent care centers. Even as solo practitioners, they consult or refer serious cases to specialists or (in the case of the specialist) to a super specialist or a university medical center. Thus, the former excuse of higher incomes as recompense for full responsibility and longer hours has evaporated; only the desire for the same high income remains. Prevalent today is the high-priced specialist associated with a for-profit hospital or partnership. These are the physicians who have the most to lose if the United States institutes universal health care. But why should doctors be entitled to incomes higher than those of other people who spend years obtaining an advanced education? Why do we persist in believing that only the prospect of a high income will attract people to medical schools? Medicine is a prestigious, intellectually challenging, and interesting profession, yielding large rewards in many non-materialistic forms.

---

[29] Robert Gumbiner, M.D., "The Doctor or the Plan: Three Case Studies," The FHP Journal of Clinical Research Vol. 4, no. 9 (Summer 1994), 56-58.

In the 1970s, I spent a six-week sabbatical studying the British Healthcare System, particularly the general practice section. I found that the majority of general practitioners at that time were in favor of the current British Healthcare System, not against it. Visiting general practitioners in various parts of England and Scotland, working in different venues including solo and group practice, in both private and government clinics, I received the distinct impression that British doctors felt they were more secure financially and could spend more time on patient care than they could prior to the establishment of the current system. In addition, they had more free time to lead normal lives, were not be bothered with bill collecting, and didn't have to practice out of their home basement offices (or their automobiles) without paid assistants. A spin-off benefit was that their patients were friendlier and more cooperative, and the monetary barriers were removed between the patient and the doctor.

In Zagreb, Croatia, I interviewed doctors working under a state system. One doctor compared his job as a physician to his father's job as a coal miner. He stated that although he made less money than his coal miner father, he much preferred being a doctor and felt fairly compensated. After all, he said, his job was less dangerous, less physically exhausting, intellectually stimulating, not boring, and conducted in a clean, air-conditioned environment. Why shouldn't he make less for being a doctor than his father did for working in the coal mines? Besides, he was educated at state expense.

Both of these anecdotes illustrate the bizarre irrationality of the way Americans regard compensation for doctors versus other professions and jobs. For national universal health care to work, we must eliminate fee-for-service medicine, a relic of the 19th century. Perhaps health care should be viewed as a public utility – regulated with regards to price and made available to everyone – with doctors, like most people in this country, paid on salary.

The objection offered by the opposition to capitated or salaried programs for doctors alleges that such an arrangement will result in lower productivity on the part of the physicians. This is contrary to the way our market-oriented democratic society operates. Most people in the United States work on a salary. How would it be if a college professor got paid more for the A and B students than C and D students? That would end in nonsense. People have varying dedication to the work ethic. The keys to productivity in our society are motivation, management, selection, and supervision. Income is a reward mechanism that seldom converts the incompetent into the competent, or the lazy person into a highly motivated worker.

Hospitals

Why should hospitals – many of which are underutilized and/or obsolete – be allowed to charge ever-higher prices for their services? Countless hospitals do not know what their true costs are, and many are not reporting accurately. Sometimes they are substituting "charges" for "costs." This is the basis for the claim that hospitals suffer large discounts to provide service for HMOs or Medicare/Medicaid. What they "charge" is what they would like to get for a service and is not necessarily based on what it costs them to provide that service; it is essentially a "wish list." For instance, if their overall costs (i.e., total cost to run the hospital, including all services divided by the number of patients at 100 percent occupancy) is $1,400/day, but their "regular" charges are set at $2,000/day, they list their costs as $2,000/day, not $1,400/day. Therefore, the payment received from organized payers such as HMOs and Medicare may actually be providing hospitals with a profit at a reasonable occupancy rate.

Hospitals claim they are losing money based upon what they would like to charge, but this never actually happens. This is a bit like a hotel claiming they are losing money because they are not getting their rack (or posted) rate from every customer, even though they are making money at rates that are discounted to travel agents, corporations, and others on a cost basis.

Under a single-payer system, hospitals would be paid a flat daily rate for each patient. It can be done. The better-run, modern hospitals will survive while the poorly-run, obsolete, or underutilized hospitals can be converted to other uses such as long-term or sub-acute care.

Blind adherence to protecting the status quo of the for-profit providers is not in the best interest of our nation and its citizens. The American Hospital Association and the AMA could play an important and vital role in creating a national health care system if they would let go of outdated ideas regarding the provision of health care on a fee-for-service, competitive basis. An essential, non-discretionary service such as health care cannot be subject solely to the objectives of competition. These organizations claim to represent the best interests of their constituents, but do they?

The collateral savings under national health insurance does not necessarily show up in the numbers because the green eyeshade boys base their fiscal analyses on everything staying the same. The savings in the cost of hospital care – which is in addition to lower utilization and the decrease in duplication of services and equipment among hospitals in our competitive system – has not been factored in. We would no longer have underutilized laboratories and imaging devices (such as scanners and X-rays) or half-empty emergency rooms in some hospitals and overflowing ERs in others (e.g., in Long Beach, California, the ER in Community Hospital, located in a higher-income area, is empty, while Memorial Hospital ER, in a low-income area, is jammed and overflowing; both are probably losing money). The savings that would result from this alone would help fund health care for everybody.

Other Players: Suppliers, Drug Companies, and Equipment Manufacturers

Industries that make enormous profits supplying the health care field, particularly those involved in pharmaceuticals and new technologies, may have much to lose if the federal government takes over the payment of health care. It's no surprise that these companies spend enormous amounts of money lobbying Congress each year to insure "favorable" conditions for their industries.

The international pharmaceutical companies are currently the most persistent, driving force affecting the rising cost of health care. They have the money, influence, and motivation to block any kind of true health care reform, particularly anything that might put a cap on their considerable profits. Unfortunately for the American people, many of the policy makers in Washington, D.C. are often ignorant of the true facts regarding health care reform, and are unduly influenced by the drug companies because of persistent lobbying efforts and campaign contributions. This influence may also include the shareholder interests of constituents and other more obscure linkages such as an increase in the value of the policy maker's stock portfolio. Pharmaceutical profits do, and will continue to, unduly influence the political reform of health care. Look at the latest Medicare prescription drug "reform" that specifically denies the federal government the right to negotiate drug prices for Medicare enrollees. What is that all about? It is not logical unless you recognize the guiding hand of drug company manipulation.

The drug companies will not attack health care reform using any kind of realistic logic; they'll use emotions – primarily fear. They will say they won't be able to develop new drugs if they face price caps (never mind that many new drugs are developed by the National Institute of Health or through grants to research institutes). They will claim that capping prices in the United States will result in lesser quality (ignoring the fact that the exact same drugs, manufactured by the same companies, are sold in Canada, Mexico, and Europe at forty to fifty percent less).

These other countries are able to sell the same drugs offered in the United States, at a lesser price, because their governments have control of the health care system. The government says to the drug company, "Here is what we are willing to pay through our national health system," and that is it. If the pharmaceutical company could not make money at that price, they would not sell the drug there. But they can and they do. This means that – if they can make a profit at the discounted prices in Canada or Mexico – they are making much larger profits at the prices charged in the United States. They are getting rich by exploiting the sick in the United States.

The companies developing new procedures and technologies are in a slightly different position, since they sell directly to doctors and hospitals rather than the end consumer. But, like the pharmaceutical companies, the senior managers of technology firms answer to investors (who want to see a profit) and use marketing to create a demand for what may be only an insignificant improvement over existing technology. Hospitals respond to marketing campaigns with the belief that this new technology is necessary to keep their physician base happy. Doctors respond to the availability of new technology by ordering tests and procedures that may not be necessary.

A system that controls the utilization of these technologies can prevent overlap, overuse, and misuse, and could reduce the overall cost of delivering quality health care in the United States. This system might include technological assessment centers (similar to those used by the National Health Care System in Great Britain) to evaluate the effectiveness of new drugs and technology. A method of sharing technological resources among multiple health care providers would control cost and improve availability.

True health care reform will require a system to evaluate the relative usefulness of new drugs and technologies. One step would be to eliminate pharmaceutical advertising to the consumer, which adds to the cost of drugs and creates a false demand for the most expensive prescription medications. Put simply, we need to modify the profit motive in exploiting the sick.

Policy Makers

Unfortunately, policy makers – legislators, civil servants, bureaucrats, and the forces that inform and influence them – represent one of the larger roadblocks to health care reform. Labor unions were one of the early driving forces behind the development of prepaid group practice, yet many unions – including the powerful AFL-CIO – refuse to endorse the idea of a single-payer national health care system. Perhaps it is because universal health care, funded through the federal government and with benefits not tied to a specific job, could dilute the role and power of labor unions. The unions, in general, have been so effective in lobbying legislature in the last thirty to sixty years that they've nearly eliminated their own jobs. They used to have to lobby for on-the-job workers' protection, and now they have that through the Occupational Safety and Health Administration (OSHA). They used to have to fight for retirement benefits, and now there are pension plans. Workers have social security; they have unemployment insurance; and they have worker's disabliity compensation. The only things left for the unions to negotiate are wages and health care.

An objective and ethical union leader should be for single-payer health care because it benefits union members. So too would an educated, logical, thoughtful politician see that universal national health care would benefit his or her constituents. Unfortunately, too many of our politicians may be motivated by self-interest (the desire to get re-elected) and influenced by the lobbies of special interest groups. The power of these lobbies must not be underestimated: in 2003, the pharmaceutical and health insurance industries alone funded 952 individual lobbyists and spent a record 141 million dollars lobbying members of Congress.[30] Too many politicians shun measures that would result in true health care reform, claiming that people simply won't pay for universal national health care through taxes or a social security deduction. Yet most individuals *already* pay for health care, either out-of-pocket or through copayments and deductibles. Polls show that the majority of Americans are in favor of the government playing

---

[30] Public Citizen's Congress Watch, "Rx R&D Myths: The Case Against the Drug Industry's R&D 'Scare Card'," (Public Citizen: 2004). Available at www.citizen.org.

a dominant role in health care. They just cannot agree on the methodology. This is no surprise, since the confusion has been devised by the opposition.

Most recently, rising health care costs are consistently cited as a major concern among citizens and employers, second only to war and foreign policy issues.[31] The best that our politicians and policy makers have come up with are ineffectual, patchwork solutions that fail to address the real problems in the system. Between the pressure of lobbyists' skewed and false information and the fear of losing votes, most of our politicians are simply unable or unwilling to take a courageous, positive position.

Wanted: A White Knight for Health Care Reform

In the course of my career, I have talked to many politicians about health care issues. Some have listened and asked intelligent questions. Many have checked their watches and let their eyes glaze over. A few of them understand the issues; some are misinformed and want to stay that way; and some of them will really listen and ask intelligent questions. But far too many have no real understanding of, and no interest in, the problems facing our health care system, nor do they have any real solutions. For health care reform to happen, our politicians have to be enlightened; they have to be intelligent, and they have to be interested in doing something. But most of all, they must have courage. Courage is universally rare in our society while, unfortunately, self-interest is prevalent. We only need one courageous person – one policy maker with the determination to fight for a universal national

---

[33] Kaiser Family Foundation, "USA Today Examines National Physician Shortage," March 3, 2005. Posted at www.kff.org.

health care system and the political savvy and power to offer health care to all Americans.

In order to change the health care system, we need what might be called a "white knight." I found a white knight once in my career, in 1967. That white knight headed the California State Assembly Health Committee. He had actually pushed through a piece of legislation mandating that the Health Department of California seek out and try to find ways of solving the problem of waste and misdirection of funds for the Medi-Cal/Medicaid program. He was one of these politicians who had courage; he also had a bad temper, and he was mad because this legislation had passed and nothing had happened.

After MediCal (Medicaid) in California had passed in 1967, I spent every month for two years contacting people in Sacramento (the state capital) because I was convinced that MediCal, under the fee-for-service system, would fail and not achieve its purpose: available, accessible, and affordable care for the poor. I had written letters, met with government officials, and testified before the State Assembly, focusing on the concept that Medicaid could not operate efficiently under the fee-for-service system. Doctors in general did not practice where the poor people lived, and most of those poor people did not have transportation to get to the doctors. Besides, they did not know how to access the system. You can't drag three sick kids on public transportation out to the suburbs to see the doctor during his or her office hours of 9:00 AM to 5:00 PM. If you work six days a week cleaning hotel rooms, you need to see the doctor in the evenings or on Sunday; you can't take time off work to suit the doctor's convenience. Besides, with no oversight of utilization, it was clear to me that fee-for-service billing would soon deplete the MediCal fund.

On one of my regular monthly visits, I was discussing this issue with my local assemblyman, expressing frustration that my proposal to enroll MediCal patients on a pilot project capitation basis was not getting consideration. It was a slow Thursday afternoon in Sacramento. He took me to see the head of the Assembly Health Committee. I gave this man a file containing all the proposals I'd made and the testimony I had given at various hearings. He took a look at it and immediately called up the head of the State Health Department, who had jurisdiction. I will never forget it. He said, "I've got a man sitting here who's made a proposal for a pilot project that looks like it makes sense. I want you to do something about this or else I'm going to the corner office." (The "corner office" referred to the governor of California, who at that time was Ronald Reagan, also a Republican.) There was a short pause, and then he said, "You can see him today? Good."

Twenty minutes later, I was sitting in front of the head of California Public Health, a man who had been ignoring me for two years. Flanked by his two chief aides, he looked at me and said "Dr. Gumbiner, I think there's been some mistake. We've reviewed your proposal and we think it has merit." Obviously, they had reviewed the proposal in the twenty minutes it took me to walk over from the legislative offices. But at least they had – finally – reviewed it. He asked me "When can you start?" It was June, so I said, "In October." I would just make it happen! His aides began to get nervous at this point and make noise. He just looked at them and said, "I'm sure we can meet that deadline."

As an aside, a couple of months after the program started, these same two aides showed up at our Long Beach office and said, "Where is the dental program?" I replied, "What dental program?" Sure enough, they had left it out of the original agreement. But thirty days later, by joining with a friend of mine who had a large dental office and experience with union capitation programs, we had our first dental program. The point is, get it started and repair it later. If Henry Ford had tried to start with the Thunderbird instead of the Model T, we would all still be walking or taking the train.

What is most important about this whole story is that I – personally – had no political influence. I hadn't made a big campaign contribution to anyone. I was just visiting my assemblyman on one of my monthly tours to Sacramento, because that is what you do when you're trying to get the government to do something. You visit your elected representative. Fortunately, my representative was willing to introduce me to the head of the Assembly Health Committee, and – also fortunately – he was available that day. Most importantly, this politician was willing to take a stand for something he believed in.

Some time after that initial meeting, I asked him how he was able to have so much influence with the State Health Department. "Well, here's how it works," he said. "The Health Department has to have the recommendation of the Assembly Health Committee to get their budget approved. So when they called me to ask about progress on their budget, I asked about progress on the Medi-Cal pilot project. It's just give and take."

That's what happens in politics. It is always about give and take. Any strong, committed politician can do for universal national health care what was done in California for Medi-Cal reform in the 1960s. The operative word is *strong*; some politicians are weak, and they do not want to take any chances. Other politicians don't want to confront anyone, or they are afraid some constituents or a wealthy supporter may be opposed, so they are not going to take action. A white knight who is really interested in health care reform could write the legislation and push it through. It just takes courage and commitment.

The two most important pieces of social legislation passed in the last century in the United States were the Social Security Act under Franklin D. Roosevelt's administration and the Medicare/Medi-Cal legislation under President Lyndon B. Johnson. Both of these men were master politicians who would not take no for an answer and knew how to push the buttons in Congress and elsewhere. Perhaps the opposition wasn't as powerful then, but now the stakes are higher. President Roosevelt and President Johnson were real "white knights," and they had plenty of vicious, determined opponents. Yet they prevailed and, ultimately, established the programs the country needed.

Chapter 7

The Cure – Basic Solutions that Work

What is missing in the current debate on universal national health care – something that a majority of Americans believe is a good idea – is any discussion of how to make it happen. We have yet to get beyond how national health care will be paid for. This should be a non-issue. We are already paying for health care that is overpriced and inadequate. *Any tax or payroll deduction for universal health care would be in place of – not in addition to – the monies individuals, employers, and the government pay now* for health care coverage.

If we can get beyond the "how is it paid for?" question, there are still thorny issues surrounding how we make it work. Most policy makers are wary of discussing the need for the government to get involved in health care. They are even more afraid of discussing just how the delivery of health care needs to be managed. Few politicians have considered the issue of re-educating health care providers, and even fewer want to discuss it. There are *three critical components* in establishing *effective* universal national health care in the United States: 1) how it is paid for, 2) how to make it work in a cost-effective manner, and 3) how to get the providers on board.

The Role of the Federal Government

Taking an incremental approach, national universal health care could be phased in gradually, starting with an expanded Medicare covering children and obstetric care. Then the age limit could be lowered from sixty-five to fifty-five to include that section of our population now most in need of health care. Next, we could merge Medicaid into Medicare, getting rid of the current wasteful overlap and state-by-state patchwork system for the poor. If all of this were accomplished, the remaining population utilizing private insurance, and available to spread the risk for the for-profit health insurance sector, would be so small that insurance companies may choose to exit the field. Everyone in the country would eventually be covered under a Medicare system providing *complete* coverage.

For this to happen, *the federal government must act as the single payer for health care,* just as it is the single payer for highway systems, clean water, and the military. Money would be collected through a payroll deduction (on the part of employees) and payroll contribution (on the part of employers), establishing a single fund and creating one large risk pool of all Americans. Yes, universal health care may require a new tax or payroll deduction. But remember, this deduction would be *in place of* the monies employers and employees pay now for health insurance, probably at a lower total cost. This key point is often ignored in the debate over how to pay for national health care. People forget that they are *already* paying – in many cases overpaying – for health care that is often inadequate or inaccessible.

Having established one large fund to pay for all health care, the government is in a better position to control the cost of that health care. Removing insurance companies from the process will reduce overall costs by as much as thirty to forty percent (the amount these companies now allocate to marketing, administration, and profit). Also, as any insurance company executive can tell you, the larger the pool, the lower the overall expenses and risk. The key is to spread the risk over the greatest number of people possible. A single pool of funds, covering 294 million people, is a very large pool indeed.

The federal government can also control costs through negotiation. Under the system I propose, the government – not the pharmaceutical companies – would be the dominant power in the health care arena. Rates for hospitals, skilled nursing facilities, prescription drugs, equipment, and supplies could all be negotiated to ensure reasonable profitability to the suppliers, without price gouging. This is what nearly every other developed-industrialized country does as a basic method of controlling the cost of health care delivery. That our country cannot even negotiate the price of prescription drugs for Medicare patients is disgraceful.

Finally, the government can further control costs by gradually introducing a "community-based" capitation rate to replace the fee-for-service "experience-based" rating system. Insurance companies currently establish monthly premiums based on what they call "experience" rating. This involves analyzing groups as to the gender of employees (because females use more health care than males), the age of the employees (because people over fifty use more health care), and finally, experience (i.e., how much health care your group used last year). If you have a group with older employees, more females, or some sick users, the insurance company is going charge a higher premium to cover everyone, or they are going to reduce the benefits.

A capitation rate or payment per person is a set amount, paid to the health care provider, per patient, to cover the agreed-upon health care expenses of that patient for a specific period.

Using a community rating to set the capitation payment, actuaries evaluate the cost to provide a benefit level to an entire community and set a single rate for everyone in that community, regardless of age, gender, or experience. This is the way prepaid group practice used to work: they established the same rate for everyone. There is a cost savings in this method because within a certain community (community being geographical, or some other form of segmentation) it is not necessary to figure out different rates for each employer group that signs up. Also, the risk is spread over a larger group and rates are based on the overall cost of delivering health care in that community.

This idea of community rather than experience rating is critical in implementing universal health care. One of the problems under the current system of experience rating is that the people least likely to be able to pay – older women on low wages – have to pay the most for health care. Community rating involves a more equitable spread of risk and mandates innovative, logical ways of organizing the delivery of health care. Community rating will not work under the current wasteful, fee-for-service system.

The other problem with our existing system is that it has developed from an odd merger of prepayment and fee-for-service. Most people "prepay" in the sense that they pay a monthly premium for health care coverage before they receive the service (and even if they do not receive service). Yet insurance companies, Medicare, and Medicaid pay out claims on what is essentially a fee-for-service basis after the service is rendered. In other words, the patient sees the doctor, who then files for reimbursement for whatever service the doctor claims to have performed. Provided that the service is covered under the patient's policy, the insurance company eventually makes a payment to the doctor. The insurance adjustor has no idea if that service was actually performed or even necessary. If there is the correct code on the claim form, they make the payment. In a very real sense, our current system of health care delivery is the worst of all worlds: prepayment based on experience rating, married to fee-for-service billing by a provider who is not responsible for the cost, and paid for by a third party with no control over that cost, which is eventually passed on to the consumer, employer, or government entity, again with no choice or control.

By changing the payment system to eventually de-emphasize or eliminate fee-for-service, we can modify the current system, which does not control costs and actually rewards excess, waste, and duplication. By paying health care providers – rather than insurance companies – a set rate, per month, per person, the government is in a much better position to control and plan for future health care costs. The providers who control delivery (unlike the insurance companies) can then manage and supply the medical care.

The Organized Provider System (OPS)

A critical component of effective universal health care has to do with how the *delivery* of health care is *organized and managed*. This – even more than having the federal government as the single payer – is a contentious issue. The majority of Americans will agree that universal national health care is a good idea. Most of them will accept that it has to be paid for through some kind of federal withholding or tax. Many will concede that the federal government is the logical choice for handling the funds. But the very idea of "managing" health care has become anathema to the American public due to the advertising and spin efforts of the AMA, the AHA, the pharmaceutical companies and the HIAA, their successors, and anyone else who has a vested interest in keeping health care expenses (and profits) as high as possible.

Let me return to one of my initial arguments: the delivery of health care does – and should – be the responsibility of health care providers. This includes doctors, dentists, nurse practitioners, and anyone who makes the choice of what is to be provided, where and when, for the patient. Few if any of these health care providers are trained in management. Yet our current system insists that doctors function as managers, performing the many financial and administrative tasks that management entails, while they simultaneously strive to provide quality care to their patients, keep up on the latest in medical developments and information, and market their services.

Envision instead a system in which health care providers work in groups run by specially trained doctor-managers. These independent Organized Provider Systems (OPS) would initially be assigned patients, by the government, based on geographic locale, and paid a flat rate per patient per month. The doctor-managers would receive these capitation payments, per head per month, from the government program, using those payments to create and maintain facilities, and pay salaries and benefits for health care personnel, while ensuring proper utilization and quality of care. Out of the fee paid by the federal government, the OPS could provide a full spectrum of care – including various forms of hospitalization, rehabilitation, preventative, and psychiatric care, and prescription drugs – with a minimal copayment from some recipients. Most importantly, the OPS would place the responsibility for delivering quality care at a reasonable cost where it belongs: on the decision makers, the health care providers.

The assignment of patients to the OPS by the government eliminates the very important need for these groups to spend time and money on marketing and enrollment. Patients could reselect their OPS on a periodic basis. The existence of multiple OPS groups in most areas would mean the OPS would have to offer quality service; if they don't, patients will switch to a different OPS. (For example, Germany's nationally funded health care program allowed individuals to switch doctors every ninety days.)

The OPS would be organized to provide the full array of health care professionals needed to give each member complete health care: medical, dental, optometry, pharmaceutical, psychiatric, and hospitalization. The capitation payment has to cover all these services, because not covering prescription drugs and preventive care would result in an incomplete vehicle, like an auto without one wheel. Organized, capitated prepayment systems have, in the past, proven to be thirty to fifty percent more cost effective than fee-for-service systems.[32]

Why should this Organized Provider System work, now, when prepaid group plans and HMOs have failed in the past? The three things that kept the more complicated group practice prepayment organizations from growing were poor marketing ability, lack of financing for facilities, and inadequate management. With my plan for the Organized Provider System (OPS), these problems will disappear.

---

[32] See previous reference to the "Report of the Legislative Analyst to the Joint Legislative Budget Committee," Analysis of the Budget Bill of the State of California for the Fiscal Year July 1, 1971 to June 30, 1972 (Sacramento, CA: California Legislature, 1971 Regular Session), 14-16.

First of all, there will no longer be a need for money spent on marketing and sales because consumers will be assigned initially to various organized provider groups. They will then have the choice of getting out of the assigned OPS and into another on a thirty-day notice. By assigning recipients to the OPS initially, money will start coming into each OPS from the day they open, solving the financing problem.

Secondly, the construction of new facilities would not be a problem because a government loan guarantee could be made available to build facilities, with architectural plans for their construction provided. Some facilities might even be pre-manufactured modular units. This means medical facilities could be built in a cost-effective manner, with financing available for construction.

Next and most importantly is the need for competent management. Trained doctor-managers should run these organizations, having acquired the education they need for recruiting, organizing, controlling, and planning. (That education, in itself, requires a plan to make it work – something I address in the next section.) From the day they open the door, each OPS will have operating income since they will have prepaid clients assigned to them; a key issue. I suggest that the OPS first secures the management, second, acquires the facility, third, recruits the doctors, and fourth, starts operations.

The OPS would collect payment from the government based on the number of individuals enrolled. Management and health care professionals would be paid on salary, with a modest profit participation based on group performance and patient satisfaction. It is possible that the OPS could be set up in a manner similar to public utilities; allow reasonable levels of profit in a controlled environment. Health care – like electricity or potable water – is a basic need. To attract talented management, some financial incentive may be necessary. The average OPS could contract with specialized hospitals or medical school-based OPS for sub-specialty service.

Some hospitals and pharmacies could continue to be run independently while contracting with local OPS on a flat, daily rate or capitation basis. Hospitals should actually be able to operate more efficiently on a capitation payment basis, as this eliminates waste and provides a predictable income for financial planning purposes.

With the OPS providing an umbrella, health care providers will be able to deliver a higher quality of care at a lower overall cost due to the consolidation of technology and management, access to a universal data bank of prescriptions and treatments, and the centralization of patient records. The OPS will also eliminate the need for individual doctors to pay for malpractice insurance. (In fact, with proper management and quality control, the instances of malpractice and cost of insurance should be reduced.)

The biggest obstacles to the successful operation of the OPS, theoretically, would be lack of financing, poor management, and excessive risk. These three problems contributed to most of the failures in the early group practice prepayment plans that the federal government sponsored in the 1970s. Today, however, since we know where the potholes are, we can avoid them. With careful planning and lessons learned from the health insurance and group practice prepayment fields, the solutions are available.

The first problem is that of risk, or excessive loss, which includes medical conditions beyond the capacity of the OPS to treat or pay for. *The answer is reinsurance.* This concept has been around for a long time and is well known to anyone involved in managing insurance companies. A reinsurance company insures risk layers over and above the primary risk covered by the basic carrier, in this case the OPS. One of the problems that start-up organizations (such as a new OPS) face is that they have little or no reserves to cover unexpected high-cost medical cases outside of their contractual service capacity, which could include hospital expenses or super-specialty services. Reinsurance paid for from a percentage of the premium would solve this problem.

The OPS has some big advantages over a health insurance company. First, the OPS is a direct service organization and provides the health care services. This allows for flexibility and innovation in providing about eighty percent of necessary services to the average patient. Next, since the OPS is ordering and selecting the outside services, they, unlike patients or claims adjusters, will know when they are being overcharged or billed for services never received by their patients, thus further reducing the risk.

The problem with obtaining reinsurance for a start-up OPS is that there are not enough people covered at first to make it profitable to write reinsurance for this group because of the inability to spread risk. And there is not enough money coming in from that particular organization to cover the reinsurer's administrative expenses for that OPS. When I was running FHP, with over a million individuals covered by the HMO plus three insurance companies, it became much easier and less expensive to obtain reinsurance the larger we became.

The answer for these start-ups is that *the federal government would act as the re-insurer, as part of the universal health plan.* By spreading the risk over 294 million people, the cost to the OPS for reinsurance should be very low. The problem would be to keep the OPS from over-reliance on the federal government's reinsurance program, that is, from not caring what costs they run up on a patient once they reached the reinsurance level.

This can be solved by a simple prorated system, with the OPS responsible for the first $100,000 in each case. Then a corridor of fifty-fifty coverage by the OPS and re-insurer for the next $100,000, then $75,000 for the re-insurer and $25,000 for the OPS for the next $100,000, and finally a cap of $300,000 total loss coverage for the OPS for each case. Thereafter, the federal government insurance would take over. This would provide a $175,000 total stop-loss for the OPS, per case. They could purchase an annual combined all-case stop-loss in addition.

The reason the OPS concept is so workable is that under this system, *each organized provider service would have an immediate income the day they opened their doors.* The federal health care program would assign the covered individuals on a prepaid basis to each OPS and eliminate the cost and time lag of marketing and enrollment (they could opt out in thirty days to join a different OPS). From the first day of operation, the OPS would have a *planned monthly income without accumulating a start-up deficit.* They could, by operating on an approved budget, begin immediately to set aside reserves for every expected loss, and pay overhead and any debt service they had accumulated for facilities and equipment.

This concept of government-funded reinsurance could also be applied to medical malpractice insurance. In addition to my earlier suggestion of getting rid of the twenty percent of doctors who are responsible for eighty percent of the malpractice claims, the federal government health plan could offer malpractice reinsurance on a participatory basis to the OPS. The economy of scale that comes from covering thousands of doctors works; I've done it.

In the staff model HMO I managed for over thirty years, we purchased coverage for approximately 400 doctors, 200 dentists, and 100 pharmacists, with a three million-dollar deductible. This may seem like a big number, but when you divide that three million by the 700 professionals, that deductible amounted to less than $5,000 per year per individual. In addition, we had our own claims prevention and adjustment system employing one full-time attorney at our corporate headquarters and a claims advisor in each of our six state regions. These people followed up on any complaint or alleged problem and corrected or settled it before it got into litigation. Problem physicians involved in multiple malpractice claims were terminated. The ability to partially self-insure, eliminate problem health care providers, and negotiate premiums resulted in huge savings and a reasonable insurance expense per doctor. Since we provided the service, there was no "tail" (i.e., no unknown claims yet to be filed against unknown doctors).

The management problem facing the OPS could be solved by training appropriate doctors in management from the beginning of their careers. Forget the legal and medical group habit of giving the management job to the least competent attorney or doctor in the group. My plan would produce an abundance of bright, capable doctor managers who prefer the managerial track from the start. As in any business, these doctor-CEOs would be the highest paid physicians in the system.

Financing facilities and operations should be easy through federal health plan financing or guarantees. The OPS eventually pays back these loans or bond issues. This has also been done before. My first FHP general hospital was financed through a $35 million bond issue, guaranteed by the State of California Health Facilities Act. Again, that was a straightforward application, involving no lobbyists and no campaign contributions; I did not even know anybody in the government.

But it was not easy. The then-treasurer of the State of California was head of this health facilities committee. Three days before my first appearance in regard to my application, I got a call from somebody who suggested I contribute to a Political Action Committee with this individual's name on it. I turned them down because I did not want to get involved with that, and I did not have the money. Of course, when I appeared before the committee, my application was turned down. I just kept appearing at each one of their monthly meetings, and finally I talked to this man's assistant and convinced him that we were what we were, a non-profit organization made up of doctors who did not have any money. At a subsequent meeting, we were approved without a problem.

Again, I must emphasize that with the system I am proposing for the OPS, operating income to reach the break-even point does not have to be built up week by week, month by month, through initial deficit financing and intensive marketing efforts, because the patients will be assigned to the OPS based on their geographic location, with the option to move to another OPS on a periodic basis. Since most patients follow the plan, not the doctor (and since most people don't have a regular doctor or know how to find one), assignment should not be a problem. To provide choice, the individual could opt out to a different OPS on a periodic basis. Most importantly, the OPS will not have the problem of having to develop income to meet their operating budget. The operating income is there from the start in the form of prepayment capitation from the federal government. The whole marketing cost and the effort it entails could be eliminated.

This is in some ways similar to a free clinic I was involved with in Mexico with the Flying Samaritans. Three doctors and two nurses arrived at a five-bed hospital late at night and lay down on the beds. In the morning, when we woke up, our patients had come in during the night and were lying on the floor. We stood up, they stood up, and the clinic was in session. No start-up time, no delays, and minimal costs. The same principle can work for the OPS: hire a doctor manager, recruit the doctors, borrow money through the government program to build pre-designed medical facilities, and install equipment that has been pre-selected and purchased through a volume discount. The construction of these facilities would be based on established criteria regarding location, or patient accessibility, and hours the center is open and available to patients. Patients are assigned the day the OPS opens its doors, and capitation payments for the first month are received before providing the services. (The possible weakness in this system would be poor management. Help in this area could be provided through a set of management criteria plus evaluation protocol, much like that used in the Military Officer Corps.)

If these OPS are set up as a type of public utility with proper oversight controls, plus a protocol for the organizational structure, and approved fiscal and accounting plans with budgets to allow for adequate reserves, this structure can be kept simple and understandable: a guaranteed plan for success. I proved that this could be done in our Guam unit. We were sponsored by the government of Guam, which helped enroll employees with a new mandatory selection of health plans by each individual and an orientation session conducted on employer time. All health care services were covered under a government-funded, prepaid capitation plan. The three elements were there: government support with minimal marketing costs, fully-equipped medical centers, and an immediate, large enrollment, spreading the risk. We supplied the management, the recruitment, the training, the systems, and controls. As an added feature, everyone was enrolled in our program unless they opted for an alternate plan – not an unusual feature of many union programs.

Of course, not everyone in the United States lives in an area with a population large enough to support the OPS; or doctors may be few and far between in poor urban communities. These areas could be served by individual doctors or smaller primary clinics affiliated with the closest OPS for specialty services. Perhaps the capitation rate could be slightly higher for the doctors serving rural and poor urban areas as a means of attracting much needed health care providers to these poorly served locales. In this model, each primary care doctor or small clinic would have a prepaid panel, which is a list of available doctors with availability to take additional prepaid patients. (An example of how this can work is the British system, which originally offered incentives of higher compensation for general practitioners over specialists and for less desirable geographic assignments.)

No matter how well-designed the system, there will, undoubtedly, be individuals who will insist on their right to go outside their assigned OPS for care or alternate opinions. These people could be given the choice of paying extra for a second tier of coverage. This second tier would be a kind of "supplemental" coverage, allowing individuals alternate choices of doctors or venues for care, with a wider level of prescription drug coverage. Coverage for this could be wrapped into the government program through higher co-pays. I would suggest a co-pay of forty percent on the first $2,000 then thirty percent of the balance for each service or prescription. Or this copayment coverage could be provided through an insurance company. There, the cost would be high because of adverse selection by the sick and a smaller spread of risk, in addition to the margin for insurance company profits.

Most importantly, everyone – adult or child, employed or unemployed – would still have a safety net of essential health care services under the basic national universal health care plan without additional charge. So if an individual chooses a high-option plan but stops paying, he or she is automatically covered under the basic plan at no additional cost. This is not the either/or of the usual two-tier coverage, but rather a "basic plan plus." Doctors outside of the system would be paid on a fee-for-service basis with a fee schedule. The patient payment of thirty to forty percent should help control waste and unnecessary duplication. Remember, this second tier would be "add-on" service, not basic care.

What I'm proposing is a national health care program, paid for by the federal government and serviced by health care professionals, and managed mostly by privately run Organized Provider Systems. The government may, initially, need to subsidize the cost of establishing the OPS through loans or supplemental payments, but that cost would be recouped quickly in savings. More importantly, effective management would guarantee a system that provides the most care to the most people for the least amount of money.

Under this system, access to health care would no longer be tied to employment. Employers would not have to spend days and weeks each year evaluating rival health insurance plans and negotiating with unions and employer/consumer groups. Doctors and other health care professionals would not have to worry about whether or not the patient is "covered," nor wade through the various benefits offered by a plethora of health plans. Nor would the doctor have to argue with the patient about their coverage:

"Go ahead, Doc, I'm covered."

"No, you are not. It's excluded."

"Who's covered – you or your husband?"

"Which plan covers your children?"

Most importantly, the barriers to accessing health care would be removed, encouraging early access to care and decreasing the need for expensive emergency care and hospitalization.

The benefits of this new program are fairly obvious to most, but not all. As a society, we benefit by having a healthier working population; the government benefits by paying less, overall, to maintain that healthier population; and employers benefit by the reduced cost and escape from the hard-to-understand, complicated health insurance business. Health care professionals will no longer have to spend hours filling out claim forms and trying to "game" the system. They can concentrate on taking care of people.

Individuals would no longer have to worry about whether or not they can access health care when they need it. They will have a choice of physicians within their assigned OPS and the option of changing to another OPS or upgrading to a second-tier, high-option program with a copayment.

A single-payer program of capitated payments eliminates the current wasteful and frustrating complication of multiple insurance plans and coverage. All patient care and information can eventually be coordinated electronically within the entire OPS system (which provides the direct service), eliminating the costly and possibly dangerous duplication of procedures and prescriptions.

As a byproduct, there will be a huge amount of valuable data available through the system for research and future planning.

This medical research can be organized and focused to develop a type of man-on-the-moon approach, which means a planned, coordinated effort by everyone involved to reach a specific objective in a stated amount of time. Add to this the possibility of establishing independent technological assessment centers within the system, which would eliminate many useless or duplicate new procedures and treatments.

Heal the Healers: Re-educating Medical Professionals.

This brings me to the most critical component in establishing effective universal health care: *the reorganization of the education of doctors and other health care professionals.* This is probably the area most in need of reform if we are to fix our existing, dysfunctional system of health care delivery and reduce our excessive health care costs.

I believe that we cannot reform health care in this country unless *we first reform the educational system for doctors.* Fee-for-service medicine provides the wrong financial incentives to doctors by encouraging the greatest volume and most expensive procedures. For national universal health care to succeed, we must look to a time when all doctors are educated within the system. I saw this when I studied Mexico's health care system. The doctors who were educated under the single-payer system did just fine; those doctors who were educated and practiced under the previous fee-for-service method often had a hard time adjusting to the new national health care program.

Most people attending medical school today will not be working under the sole practitioner, fee-for-service model in the future. Today, less than twenty-five percent of doctors in the United States are in solo practice. The rest are working in medical groups or on salary at hospitals or clinics. In addition, fifty percent or more of today's medical students are women, who often prefer more regular hours and the less stressful life of a salaried physician. Many women, and men, want more time for normal family and interpersonal relations. Those doctors who are willing to put in long hours providing patient care do not really want to spend their time on administration and paperwork; they want to practice medicine. Since patients rarely pay the doctor directly, the doctor must submit myriad forms to various insurance companies and Medicare/Medicaid for reimbursement. Medical education designed to prepare doctors for the multifaceted role of doctor/entrepreneur/administrator simply does not exist in today's world, nor should it.

The current medical educational curriculum is outdated on a number of levels. Mainly, it emphasizes the techno-scientific approach to medicine. Later, sometime during their residency training, some physicians acquire what I call the "Gold Cadillac Complex." They may come into their residencies with intellectual curiosity about medicine and a desire to be a caregiver, but they leave with the new objective of joining the affluent society. Perhaps they want to emulate private attending physicians. Maybe they spent their time in training commiserating with each other about how they are all working long hours for low wages compared with some of their peers in other fields. The fee-for-service model may provide a "financial light at the end of the tunnel" for them. Not all go through this transformation, but enough do to be a problem.

For multiple reasons, we have far more specialists and super specialists than primary care doctors in this country. This situation results from the attraction of income, prestige, and the decrease in stress by narrowing the field of knowledge. Most of the teachers in medical schools are themselves specialists who may have spent very little time in a clinical practice.

They may go from a residency to a fellowship to a teaching position. There may be little emphasis on care giving, and heavy emphasis on procedure.

I do not believe that all graduates of medical school should become clinicians. I have been in this field a long time, and I can tell you, not all doctors are good at dealing with patients. Some doctors are better at research and others are better at management. We need to provide a new type of training program for doctors, *offering a choice of one of three tracks: a clinical track, a research track, and a management track.* This would give the emerging doctor more choices for appropriate career development, and a better personality fit to help them avoid future boredom and frustration.

Medical schools should also look at providing post-graduate re-education to doctors interested in switching to a management, research, or a clinical track. The average, young medical student has little idea of what is in store for him or her in future years of practice. Unfortunately, doctors today do not have many options in terms of career growth or change.

After my father's graduation from the University of Chicago Rush Medical School in 1918, he started as a general practitioner, advanced after a few years to "Special Interest in Internal Medicine" and then on to further specialization within that field. This was before the proliferation of residency programs spawned by the GI Bill after World War II (which incidentally paid doctors at government expense while they were in residency training).

In my father's day, a doctor could advance to a specialty, doing something new and different at several stages along the way of a fifty year career. Today, the doctor finishes his or her residency, begins practice in a specialty and, for the most part, does the same thing for forty or fifty years. No wonder they seek their rewards in materialistic acquisitions and activities. I found that many doctors who had been practicing clinical medicine for ten or fifteen years welcomed the chance to branch out into other areas through our management training program. Few, if any, of the doctor-managers we trained ever wanted to go back to clinical medicine. Health care professionals with ten or twenty years in the field can, with additional education, provide the management needed to run effective Organized Provider Systems.

We also need to attract a more diverse group of students to medical schools. Part of the problem in our current system is that many people enter medical school with the wrong motivation. They may be motivated by a need for prestige or a desire for an affluent lifestyle or both, or they may have a scientific or technological orientation rather than a dedication to providing care. Perhaps they are in medical school only because they come from a long line of doctors or an upper-middle-class background.

Medical schools may also be attracting only those students who lack family obligations and have the ability to pay the tuition or can pay back thousands of dollars in student loans. This kind of financial situation automatically limits the diversity and talent of those being trained as doctors. One result is that we end up with a limited supply of physicians, mostly white and middle-class, skewed towards high paying specialties and practicing primarily in affluent areas. Good primary care physicians willing to work in rural and poor urban areas are in short supply.

The answer is to attract the best and brightest from all ethnic groups and all walks of life by removing the financial barriers to attending medical schools and modifying the inflated financial rewards currently held out to doctors. The first part of this solution is relatively easy: pay qualified people to attend medical school (and nursing school, pharmacology school, etc.). By this I mean pay for tuition and books and offer a reasonable salary while in school. Anyone with the inclination, intelligence, and aptitude could afford to become a doctor or nurse under this system.

This plan is not as far-fetched as you might think. During World War II, ninety percent of medical school students had their tuition and books, plus a per diem allowance and a salary, paid by the military. If the military could do this during a major war, I am sure the federal government can do it in peacetime. In reality, having the government underwrite medical training may be the *only* way to insure an adequate supply of physicians. We are facing a potential shortage of 85,000 to 200,000 physicians in this country by the year 2020.[33] It is a myth that anyone can go to medical school if they want to; many people cannot get past financial hardships or family obligations to attend eight years of university and another three to five years of specialty training.

By educating doctors and other providers of health care at the government's expense, an obligation could be created to spend some time in high-need areas upon completion of schooling. More people would be attracted to the primary care field, since all doctors would be paid the same. Perhaps the primary care doctor's income could be more than the specialist's, as in the British system. This might reduce the problem of different levels of prestige by specialty (and perhaps eliminate the dismissive, "Oh, you're just a family practitioner" as well).

Most importantly, basing medical school admission on competitive exams and aptitude (rather than the ability to pay)

---

[33] Kaiser Family Foundation, "USA Today Examines National Physician Shortage," March 3, 2005. Posted at www.kff.org.

should insure a better end result: humanistic care givers. The current system, in general, selects candidates for medical school based on ability to survive financially and grade point average, neither being a measure of who will be an effective caregiver or physician. The problem is that the people with high grade point averages are often those who prefer the less interactive pursuits of study and research rather than dealing with people. There is an old saying that sometimes the "A" students end up working for the "C" students because the "C" students may be more action- and people-oriented.

Redesigning the medical education system to attract people from all walks of life and steering them toward one of three tracks (clinical, research, or management) should increase the number of doctors as well as the efficiency of the health care system overall. The nonsensical idea that people will not apply for medical school unless they can make a fortune is just that: nonsense. In other countries – where the doctors actually work within a government-run system – there are an overwhelming number of applicants for medical schools. Health care is an interesting, rewarding, and respected profession, offering great personal satisfaction to people with altruistic ideals and intellectual curiosity.

It is also nonsense to think we will end up with "too many" doctors under this system. The supply of doctors will be much easier to regulate if the government is paying for their training. The key to making national universal health care work lies in controlling the supply with regards to the number of doctors, their qualifications, and what specialties and geographic locations these doctors choose. If you train an ample supply of doctors, then you have enough doctors to staff the system without anyone having to work sixty or eighty hours a week. Because the practice of medicine will be less stressful, and medical education will be paid for by the federal system, doctors won't expect astronomical salaries. Working in teams under less stress will also mean fewer mistakes, more thoughtful decision-making, more time for preventive care, and a better lifestyle for providers.

With incomes at reasonable levels, the system can support all the doctors we need, as primary care physicians, specialists, and super specialists are created. It is a myth that producing more doctors will create more care, more utilization, and higher health care costs. This happens only under the fee-for-service system, through which doctors can manufacture additional care, visits, and procedures for a financial incentive. What will be created under a capitated system are more options for doctors. Doctors can be trained for clinical, research, or management positions, according to their personalities and aptitudes. Clinicians can be distributed more effectively, by specialty and geographically, based upon need. For example, we don't have nearly enough geriatricians, given the graying of America. According to the Alliance for Aging Research, the nation currently has less than half the geriatricians needed, and by 2030, we may have less than one-third.[34] Perhaps everybody would be better off if the pediatricians, at the age of fifty, were required to retrain as geriatricians. Since we are producing fewer children and living longer, this might freshen up the doctors' professional lives and make more sense in allocating personnel to specialties.

In the Cuban system, where they produce four times the number of doctors that the population needs, the average doctor spends only two or three days a week in patient care and the balance of his or her time in preventive medicine, such

---

[34] Bob Moos, "Aging baby boomers outpace trained doctors," The Dallas Morning News, September 2, 2005. Available at www.tallahassee.com.

as well-baby clinics, prenatal and postpartum clinics, health education, hypertension, diabetes, or other chronic disease prevention. So what is the worst that could happen in the United States? Perhaps so many people will apply for medical school that only the best, brightest, most caring people are admitted, and those people will have the time to really practice medicine. That would not be a bad problem to have.

Glossary

Adverse Selection: A situation in which, according to insurance company jargon, only the high risk enroll in the insurance program, resulting in higher claim rates and thus causing excessive financial losses.

AHIP (America's Health Insurance Plans): AHIP is the national trade association representing nearly 1,300 member companies providing health insurance or HMO coverage to more than 200 million Americans.

AHA (American Hospital Association): Founded in 1898, the AHA has close to 43,000 individual and organizational members, representing and serving all types of hospitals and health care networks.

AMA (American Medical Association):   Founded in 1847, the AMA is the leading professional association of, and advocate for, more than 650,000 physicians in the United States.   In the early part of the twentieth century, the AMA was instrumental in creating and implementing standards for physician education.

Capitation: One payment per head. This comes from the Latin root *capit*, meaning *head*. A prepayment for health care services made each month for each contract; i.e., individual.

COBRA (Consolidated Omnibus Reconciliation Act): A government program that mandates health insurance coverage for those who have become unemployed or change jobs. Although it mandates benefits, it does not regulate premium rates so many individuals are priced out of this market. This is another "Band Aid" solution.

Co-Pay: An amount paid by the patient at the time of service, in addition to their monthly premium payment to the insurance company or HMO. The co-pay may be stated as a set amount or as a percentage of the total charged by the provider.

Deductible: The amount of money that must be paid by the individual covered by an insurance policy before an insurance policy begins payment. This can vary from $100 per day in a hospital to $2,000 total, per case, and can be per illness or per year, per individual or per contract.

Exclusions and Limitations: These are usually things that the plan will not cover or will cover only partially. It is very important to know what the exclusions and limitations are. The most usual *exclusion* is obstetrical coverage; some plans can totally exclude coverage for care received out of their service area or for certain procedures or illness (e.g., experimental treatment, some unproven drugs). Even Medicare excludes care outside the United States. *Limitations*, on the other hand, indicate the maximum the insurance policy will pay for a particular service. For example, it may limit the pharmaceuticals covered to generic equivalents, or it may limit how much will be paid for a particular procedure.

GHAA (Group Health Association of America): This was the original prepaid group practice association. The Group Health Association of America eventually merged into an association with the HIAA and became a type of representation for all types of health care coverage.

HIAA (Health Insurance Association of America): This was an association of most of the major companies that provided health insurance. It has subsequently been merged with Health Plans of America, the former national organization for HMOs.

HMO (Health Maintenance Organization): A term coined by Dr. Paul Ellwood and adopted in conferences held in Jackson Hole, Wyoming. It originally referred mostly to the group practice pre-payment organizations, but later expanded to include IPAs and some insurance company products that posed as HMOs. Legislation in 1973 legitimized the HMO concept.

IPA (Independent Practice Association): This outgrowth of the HMO benefited doctors who were not associated with group practice prepayment organizations but, by forming an IPA, where allowed to sign up and receive payment on a capitation basis or some other modified fee-for-service basis. In return, the capitation limited their fees but not the utilization. Individual physicians were loosely associated with the IPA organization, which supposedly provided some quality control and a list of participating doctors.

Indemnity Insurance: A policy for which an insurance company indemnifies or agrees to pay a set amount for each procedure.

Medicare: A program created during the Lyndon Johnson Administration, on July 30, 1965, to provide healthcare for people over age sixty-five. The federal government, through Social Security, is the universal single payer. In most instances Medicare shops out claims management to the claims departments of insurance companies. Medicare is a federally funded program which pays providers directly for fee-for-service care based upon a fee schedule, but it does not control volume or utilization.

Medicaid (called MediCal in California): A program to provide health care for poor and low-income Americans, Medicaid is a matching program with the states, not a totally federally funded program like Medicare. The federal government matches the money that the states put up for their programs. Originally, states were required only to provide doctor and hospital care. In the more affluent states, they have added services such as prescription drug coverage, dental, long term care, preventive services, and psychiatric services.

PPO (Preferred Provider Organization): Through a loosely held arrangement with an insurance company or IPA, the only obligation of the member doctors is an agreement to discount their inflated fee-for-service schedule. In return, they are listed as available doctors, thus saving the doctors marketing costs but offering no control over utilization.

Premium: The amount of money paid monthly for each individual covered under a health insurance plan.

SCHIP (State Children's Health Insurance Program): A program created under the Clinton Administration to provide care for children of low-income families. This is also a state matching program: the federal government matches what each state pays out annually. Many of the states simply rolled SCHIP into Medicaid; in California it became an insurance company product that attempts to charge poor people a monthly reduced premium for each child – California has considerable money left on the table because even a small monthly premium is too much for most of these families to pay.

Single-Payer: A system in which all fees are paid by one source.

Socialized Medicine: A system in which doctors are employed by the government on salary. The government owns and provides all healthcare facilities and equipment, and citizens may be automatically covered. A current example is our military hospital system, where Army and Navy doctors are paid on government salary and work in hospitals built and administered by the government. The Veteran's Administration is another example of a socialized system.

Stop Loss: A system in which people may continue to get the services but do not make additional payments. In other words, for the consumer, a stop loss is when they pay up to a certain amount, e.g. $5 or $10, for prescriptions and the plan pays for the rest. A stop loss for the insurance company is when the insurance company pays a specific amount, say for a pregnancy, and the patient pays the rest.

Utilization: The volume, amount, and extent of care provided.

Appendix A: The Doctor or the Plan?

A research report, *"The Doctor or the Plan: A Test of Family Priorities"* was published in the Blue Cross Journal *INQUIRY*, Volume VI, Number 2, 1968, written by Shirley Rich and Milton I. Roemer, M.D., Professor of the Department of Public Health, UCLA.

This article described a situation where the discontinuing of services by one of the satellite clinics of FHP forced a decision by the individuals covered through the FHP program: 1). To continue with a personal physician of their own selection with whom they were familiar, but without the FHP insurance protection; or 2). To stay with the FHP program but change doctors and medical centers.

Of 203 families, 140 (69 percent) chose to abandon their family doctors at the satellite clinic and retain their health plan membership. This suggests that the prepayment for medical care took precedence over free choice of doctor in the decisions of most families.

A follow-up article on the same subject appeared in *The FHP Journal of Clinical Research*, Volume IV, Issue 8, Winter 1994 entitled: "The Doctor or The Plan: Three FHP Case Studies".

The first study in this article involved the physicians of a network of independently contracted community-based fee-for-service physicians and the San Pedro Community Hospital where the parties were unable to reach an agreement to renew their contracts. FHP subsequently contracted with a different hospital, Bay Harbor Hospital, five miles away with a new primary and specialty care physician network. In this case the patients were all covered under Medicare and could maintain that basic coverage with the same doctors and hospital but less benefits. They had three options; continue with FHP and move to a new hospital and new group of doctors; disenroll from FHP and continue their services through their same primary care physicians and San Pedro Hospital and pay for the deductibles, copayments and uncovered services or disenroll from FHP to basic Medicare and buy "Medigap" coverage. FHP retained 73 percent of these Medicare members and lost 27 percent.

The next case was in Phoenix, Arizona in 1987. There again, an IPA network of doctors believed that if they cancelled their contract with FHP, Inc. the members would drop the plan and stay with them as fee-for-service patients covered under Medicare and Medigap.

Of FHP's 12,000 Senior Plan Medicare members in Phoenix, Arizona, 9,600 or 80 percent stayed with FHP and moved to new delivery plans changing both doctors and hospitals. They chose to retain the plan despite the fact that FHP's network had been reduced from four hospitals to just two hospitals and that the physician network had been changed.

The *FHP Journal of Clinical Research*, Volume IV, Issue 9, Summer 1994, published a Letter to the Editor summarizing three additional case studies. Again, a significant number of the people involved in these studies were individual members who had self-selected the FHP Medicare Senior Plan and had alternate coverage available through Medicare.

The first case involved 6,000 members who were being serviced by a large medical group in Southern California contracting with FHP. FHP terminated the contract with the group because of the inability to reach a satisfactory future agreement. Approximately 5,600 people of the 6,000 members, or 93 percent, stayed with FHP.

Case 2: 1991, the hospital for the FHP Torrance/Beach Cities Plan terminated its contract with FHP. Here again, this involved 1,142 Senior Plan members who were entitled to regular Medicare coverage. 96.3 percent elected to stay with FHP and transferred to a new North Torrance/Bay Harbor Plan, changing hospitals and doctors.

Case 3: December 1991 FHP terminated its provider contract for a Southern California plan. The plan consisted of 1,815 Senior Plan members and 1,380 Commercial Plan members. Following the contract termination, approximately 72 percent of the seniors remained with FHP.

These seven documented cases each in a different environment and venue, are important in dispelling the myth that patients will follow the doctor and/or local hospital not the plan. Although inertia could play a factor, it could cut both ways; i.e., stay with the doctor or with the plan. Probably the most overriding, logical reason for the absence of patient loyalty to the doctor is the fact that a majority of individuals who are financially covered for health care do not have a primary care doctor or may use hospital ER and ambulatory urgent care facilities. The extensive use of specialists and sub-specialists and lack of availability of primary care physicians accentuates the lack of a relationship between a patient and family doctor.

It appears that these examples provide more evidence that members of a health plan will follow the health plan not the individual doctor or the hospital.

Appendix B: Recommended Reading

CONSUMER ISSUES
2006

Matt Bai. "Health Care is not an Issue to Tinker With." *West Lost Angeles Times,* January 29, 2006.

Susan Brink. "Good Medical Care? It's a toss-up." *Los Angeles Times*, March 20, 2006.

Joel Havemann. "Treatment Plan for Healthcare will be Self-Help." *Los Angeles Times,* February 1, 2006.

Evan Halper. "Benefits Tab see as Major Fiscal Drag." *Los Angeles Times,* February 18, 2006.

Sarah Lueck. "Health Spending Likely to Outpace Economy's Growth." *Wall Street Journal,* February 22, 2006.

2005

Kathy M. Kristof. "Long-term Care Policies Carry No Rate Guarantees." *Los Angeles Times,* January 30, 2006.

Denise Gellene. "New Cancer Drugs are Driving up Cost of Care." *Los Angeles Times,* May 14, 2005.

Sarah Lueck. "Seeking Insurance, Individuals Face Many Obstacles." *Wall Street Journal,* May 31, 2005.

Vanessa Fuhrmans. "Patients Give New Insurance Mixed Reviews." *Wall Street Journal,* June 14, 2005.

Staff. "New Help Making Sense of Medical Research." *Wall Street Journal,* June 15, 2005.

Rob Stein, for the *Washington Post.* "Americans Have Reason to be Sick: Healthcare Costs, Error Rates Highest in U.S., Survey Finds." *Honolulu Advertiser,* November 5, 2005.

2002 - 2004

·Laura Landro. "Consumers Need Health-Care Data." *Wall Street Journal,* January 29, 2004.

Hillary Rodham Clinton. "Now Can We Talk About Health Care?" *The New York Times,* April 18, 2004.

David Wessel. "Health Spending: How Much is Too Much?' *Wall Street Journal,* January 9, 2003.

Lucette Lagnado. "Uninsured and Ill, a Woman is Forced to Ration Her Care." *Wall Street Journal,* November 12, 2002.

DELIVERY SYSTEMS
2002 - 2006

Paul Krugman (syndicated columnist). "VA: A Model for National Health Care." *Long Beach Press-Telegram,* January 30, 2006.

David Lazarus. "State Must Lead the Way." *San Francisco Chronicle,* January 18, 2004.

Nancy Sokoler Steiner. "Can Universal Care Cure State's Ills?" *The Jewish Journal of Greater Los Angeles,* June 18, 2004.

Sarah Lueck. "National Coalition on Health Care Report Urges Universal Health Care." *Wall Street Journal,* July 21, 2004.

Vanessa Fuhrmans. "Health Insurer to Target Scans for Cost Cuts." *Wall Street Journal,* August 19, 2004.

Steve Lohr. "Kaiser the Future of American Health Care?" *New York Times,* October 31, 2004.

Gina Kolata. "Program Coaxes Hospitals to See Treatments Under Their Noses." *New York Times,* December 25, 2004.

"Proposal of the Physicians' Working Group for Single-Payer National Health Insurance." *The Journal of the American Medical Association,* August 13, 2003.

Laura Landro. "Dose of Prevention: Six Prescriptions to Ease Rationing in U.S. Health Care." *Wall Street Journal,* December 22, 2003.

Marcia Angell. "The Forgotten Domestic Crisis." *New York Times,* October 13, 2002.

HEALTH INDUSTRY ISSUES
2006

"Physician, Heal Thy Country." *The Atlantic Monthly,* January 2006.

Lisa Girion. "Medical Ethics Reform Urged." *Los Angeles Times,* January 25, 2006.

Reuters News Service. "Primary Care Reforms are Urged." *The Wall Street Journal,* January 31, 2006.

2005

Rick Lyman. "Florida Offers a Bold Stroke to Fight Medicaid Costs." *New York Times,* January 23, 2005.

Sarah Lueck. "Surging Costs for Medicaid Ravage State, Federal Budgets." *Wall Street Journal,* February 7, 2005.

Rachel Emma Silverman. "New Services Cater to Affluent Patients." *Wall Street Journal,* February 9, 2005.

Barnaby J. Feder. "A Parts Supplier to an Aging Population." *New York Times,* March 26, 2005.

David E. Rosenbaum. "Medicare Outlook Called Direr than Social Security's." *New York Times,* March 24, 2005.

Tim Weiner. "A New Call to Arms: Military Health Care." *New York Times,* April 14, 2005.

Jia-Rui Chong. "Study Sees Shift in ER Care." *Los Angeles Times,* April 15, 2005.

Danny Hakim and Jeremy W. Peters. "Shares of GM Tumble on Issue of Health Care." *New York Times,* April 15, 2005.

Lisa M. Sodders. "Nursing Shortage to Get Worse." *Long Beach Press-Telegram,* April 18, 2005.

Christi Parsons. "Lawmakers Target Bad Doctors." *Chicago Tribune,* May 1, 2005.

Martin Miller. "Life Changes for Death-Care Firms." *Chicago Tribune,* May 2, 2005.

Reed Abelson. "States and Employers Duel Over Who is to Pay the Bills for Health Insurance." *New York Times,* May 6, 2005.

Robert Pear. "States Proposing Sweeping Change to Trim Medicaid." *New York Times,* May 9, 2005.

Anna Wilde Mathews. "Worrisome Ailment in Medicine: Misleading Journal Articles." *Wall Street Journal,* May 10, 2005.

Vanessa Fuhrmans. "Health Insurers' New Target." *Wall Street Journal,* May 31, 2005.

Paul Krugman (syndicated columnist). "One Nation, Still Uninsured." *Long Beach Press-Telegram,* June 14, 2005.

Melissa Healy. "Wary, and Weary, of Drug Ads." *Los Angeles Times,* June 20, 2005.

Lisa Girion. "How Much for That Brain Scan? Hospitals Reveal Prices." *Los Angeles Times,* July 2, 2005.

Lindsey Tanner (Associated Press Medical Writer). "Not What the Doctor Ordered." *Long Beach Press-Telegram,* July 13, 2005.

Robert Jablon (Associated Press). "Health Care in 'Death Spiral'." *Orange County Register,* August 4, 2005.

Harrison Sheppard. "Health Care Help From the State?" *Long Beach Press-Telegram,* August 15, 2005.

2004

Robert Tomsho. "Research Conflicts Go Undisclosed." *Wall Street Journal,* July 12, 2004.

Vanessa Fuhrmans. "Attacking Rise in Health Costs, Big Company Meets Resistance." *Wall Street Journal,* July 13, 2004.

William J. Holstein. "The Missing Rivalry in Health Care." *New York Times,* August 15, 2004.

Debora Vrana. "Health Insurance Costs Jump 11.2%." *Los Angeles Times,* September 10, 2004.

Ricardo Alonso-Zaldivar. "Medicare's Troubles May Be Sleeping Giant." *Los Angeles Times,* December 20, 2004.

2002 - 2003

Vita Reed. "Rising Health Costs Raise Tough Questions." *Orange County Business Journal,* January 2003.

Joseph B. Treaster. "To Insurers, A Long, Free Ride is Looking Risky." *New York Times,* August 9, 2003.

Vicki Kemper. "National Health Care Plan Touted." *Los Angeles Times,* August 9, 2003.

Don Lee. "Health Insurance Costs Surge." *Los Angeles Times,* September 6, 2002.

Bruce Bradley (GM Health Plans). "The Coming Crash in Health Care." *Fortune,* October 14, 2002.

INSURANCE FOR THE ELDERLY
2003 - 2006

Vanessa Fuhrmans. "Many Seniors Do The Math and Decide Not To Sign Up For The Drug-Benefit Plan." *Wall Street Journal*, February 21, 2006.

Sarah Rubenstein. "Health Insurance Often Rejects 'Near Elderly'." *Wall Street Journal*, February 21, 2006.

Jane E. Allen. "A Prescription for Injury." *Los Angeles Times*, March 10, 2003.

INTERNATIONAL HEALTH CARE ISSUES
2003 - 2005

Jeanne Whalen and Vera Sprothen. "German Curbs on Drug Costs Rile Big Brands." *Wall Street Journal*, May 2, 2005

Richard Marosi. "Healthcare is Migrating South of the Border." *Los Angeles Times*, August 2005.

Kirstin Downey. "A Hefty Dose to Swallow: The Rising Cost of Health Care in the U.S. Gives Other Countries an Edge in Keeping Jobs." *Washington Post Weekly*, March 15-21, 2004.

Clifford Krauss. "Canada Looks for Ways to Fix Its Health Care System." *New York Times*, September 12, 2004.

John Schmid. "Germans Turn Up Nose at a Dose of 'Reform'." *International Herald Tribune,* January 28, 2003.

POLITICS OF HEALTH CARE
2002 - 2006

Peter G. Gosselin. "Health Plan to Revive Debate." *Los Angeles Times,* January 23, 2006.

Richard Alonso-Zaldivar. "States Resurrect Topic of Medical Care." *Los Angeles Times,* November 13, 2005.

Jonathan Weisman. "Sick About Health Care Costs." *Washington Post Weekly,* June 7-13, 2004.

Ronald Brownstein. "Democrats Focus on Health Care For All." *Los Angeles Times,* February 24, 2003.

Robert Pear. "Alarm Again Sounds on U.S. Health Care." *International Herald Tribune,* November 21, 2002.

Appendix C: Published Works of Robert Gumbiner, M.D.

BOOKS

FHP: The Evolution of a Managed Care Health Maintenance Organization 1955-1992. Berkeley: Bancroft Library, University of California, Berkeley, 1995.

The HMO - Putting It All Together. St. Louis: Charles Mosby & Company, 1975.

ARTICLES

"Keep It Simple: Cover Prescription Drugs Through Medicare." *Press-Telegram*, August 10, 2003.

"HMO Legislation in Fantasyland." *Press-Telegram*, June 23, 2002.

"Medicare Should Cover Prescription Drugs." *Press-Telegram*, August 12, 2001.

"Take A Closer Look at Bush, Gore Prescription Drug Plan." *Press-Telegram*, October 8, 2000

"How Much is Health Care Worth to You?" *Press-Telegram*, March 19, 2000

"Drug Coverage Under Medicare Would Save Money in the Long Run." *Press-Telegram*, July 4, 1999

"FHP, Pacificare Plans Make Poor Match." *Modern Healthcare*, February 2, 1998

"Shift to Managed Care." *Press-Telegram*, April 22, 1997.

"Defending the HMOs." *Press-Telegram*, February 9, 1997.

"Like It or Not, National Health Insurance is Almost Here." *Press-Telegram*, August 4, 1996.

"A Contrarian View." *Directors' Monthly* (December 1995).

"Perspectives of an HMO Leader." *Inquiry: The Journal of Health Care Organization, Provision and Financing* (Fall 1994).

"The Yap Dispensary Program: Organizational Structures for Improving Patient Care." *FHP Journal of Clinical Research* (Summer 1994).

"Future of HMOs Depends on Quality Management." *FHP Journal of Clinical Research II*, no. 2 (1991).

"HML Prior Authorization Plan Cuts Hospital Bed Days by 28%." Presentation at the 1979 GHAA Group Health Institute.

"Selection of a Health Maintenance Organization."
Personnel Journal (August, 1978).

"Management & Marketing in Health Care." *California Medicine* (June, 1973).

"Doctors Can Do Well With Capitation Payments."
Medical Economics (November, 1972).

"The Doctor or the Plan - A Test of Family Priorities."
Blue Cross Association Inquiry (1969).

"Interviewing Prospective Group Physicians." *Medical Economics.* (1966).

"How I Interview would-be Associates." *Medical Economics* (September, 1965).